THE GRACE OF CANCER

THE GRACE OF CANCER

LESSONS IN HUMILITY AND GREATNESS

VERONICA VILLANUEVA

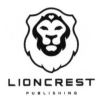

LIONCREST
PUBLISHING

THE GRACE OF CANCER

Lessons in Humility and Greatness

ISBN   978-1-5445-0793-4 *Hardcover*

978-1-5445-0792-7 *Paperback*

978-1-5445-0791-0 *Ebook*

For my readers and for myself.

CONTENTS

*"Rock bottom became the solid foundation
on which I rebuilt my life."*

—J.K. ROWLING

Sisu (n.)

*Extraordinary determination, courage, and resoluteness in
the face of extreme adversity. An action mindset that enables
individuals to reach beyond their present limitations, take
action against all odds, and transform barriers into frontiers.
An integral element of Finnish culture, and also a universal
capacity that we all share.*

Scream, cry, break down, but get up! We, the brave people
of *sisu*, do not give up! I wrote this book for *you*, my brave
friend. This is an invitation for you to find your courage
to choose TO LIVE! Fight, and push yourself, because the
reward of discovering your authentic self and true meaning in your life is your true reason for being part of this
beautiful world. Find your "why?"

True greatness is born in moments when you think you can't go on, but you keep going. Oh, how tempting it is to take the easy route—to give up—but, my friend, *breathe*. Inhale, and as you exhale, say these words: "One step at a time, I can get through this because I am strong and resilient."

According to Emilia Lathi, *sisu* begins where perseverance and grit end, so I am here alive to tell you that this darkness will bring you your brightest light, which will illuminate the world.

—VERONICA VILLANUEVA

DISCLAIMER

The information in this book pertains to the author's personal experience and should not be taken as medical advice. Please consult with a doctor before making changes to your treatment protocol.

A LETTER TO MY READERS

"Opportunity often comes disguised in the form of misfortune or temporary defeat."

—NAPOLEON HILL

On September 23, 2016, I rushed to the emergency room unable to breathe. The doctors removed 1.6 liters of fluid, enough to fill a large water bottle, from my right lung and found tumors that had metastasized on my chest, pelvis, and abdomen. They diagnosed me with "incurable" metastatic stage 4 lung cancer. Radiation and chemotherapy were not an option because the cancer had already spread, and according to my oncologist, the cancer's next target would be my beautiful brain.

Naturally, after hearing this devastating diagnosis, my next question was, "How long do I have to live?"

My doctors told me stage 4 patients could usually expect to live six months. I heard the death sentence they gave me, but all I could think was, *these doctors do not know who they're talking to or what I am capable of achieving!*

The statistics meant nothing to me—they were only numbers. I knew my own strength, and I believed that by taking responsibility for myself, I could beat the cancer. I had done the damage to my body that had caused the disease, and that gave me hope for one simple reason: it meant I also had the power to heal and reverse it.

MASTERING AND UNDERSTANDING CANCER

"There is, he said, only one good, that is, knowledge, and only one evil, that is, ignorance."

—SOCRATES

Despite what my doctors told me, I felt it in my bones that the cancer invading my body would be a short-term problem. There was no f--king way I would relinquish to this disease. I felt so determined to live, I did not even cry when I heard the diagnosis. Crying would have only added to my chronic sadness, which contributed to me getting sick in the first place.

When I looked back at this period in my life, I realized I had created the disease in my body by experiencing years of sadness, suppression, guilt, loneliness, and stress. I had allowed those toxic, negative emotions to fester for too long, so I decided to change my outlook and take responsibility for my actions.

I want to be clear, however, that responsibility is different from blame. Taking responsibility empowers you to change your circumstances, whereas blame causes nothing but negative emotions like guilt. You can react to your prognosis as a victim by blaming yourself and asking questions like, "Why did this happen to me?" or "What did I do wrong to deserve being punished with cancer?"

Instead, empower yourself by responding to the news with a positive mindset. Ask, "What lessons am I supposed to learn from this?" We tend to automatically assume the worst about our situations, but that tendency is counterproductive. Do not blame yourself for your disease, and do not think of it as a punishment.

Life is messy. Real life includes pain, suffering, and fear, not only joy, happiness, and excitement. These emotions are the admission we pay to participate in life, so avoiding them entirely means choosing not to live. We'll have plenty of time to not feel any emotions—when we are dead! Instead, accept responsibility, and if you've allowed yourself to dwell on negative emotions for too long, pivot and move forward. To heal, you need to adopt a positive mindset and truly, deeply believe that the world is better with you in it.

Science and spirituality both support the idea that a strong connection exists between the mind and body. Physics asserts that our perception forms our reality. Neuroscience tells us our thoughts influence our biochemistry. Spirituality says that life doesn't happen to us, it unfolds from us. The mind and body affect each other in every way, and if we are not healthy mentally and spiritually, we cannot be healthy physically.

Once I knew about these connections, I wholeheartedly believed I had the power to undo the damage I had inflicted on myself. I had two choices: to become a victim of cancer or to heal my body and become the absolute best version of myself. I chose the obvious—to be the Grace of Cancer—**to live**!

FINDING PURPOSE

"There is one quality which one must possess to win, and that is definiteness of purpose, the knowledge of what one wants, and a burning desire to possess it."

—NAPOLEON HILL

WHAT IS CANCER?

Cancer occurs when cells act abnormally. Normal cells eventually die when they go through a process called apoptosis. Cancer cells, however, do not go through apoptosis and do not die. These cells instead grow faster, start dividing, and spread to different parts of the body where they may form tumors. When cancer cells spread from where they originated to different parts of the body, they are said to have metastasized.

Cells may begin to act abnormally due to an overload of chemicals, toxins, and other stressors, like emotional turmoil. When our bodies are exposed to toxins, diseases eventually develop, and normal cells transform into cancer cells.

Cancer cells can make their own blood supply for nourishment to grow and spread. Like a parasite, cancer robs resources from the body and, over time, can overwhelm the body. This is called "wasting away."

Cancer can attack different parts of the body, including the glands, bones, organs, blood, and the lymphatic system, and acts differently depending on its location.

Cancer can form three types of tumors:

- **Carcinomas:** These tumors grow in an organ that usually secretes fluids. For example, lung tissue secretes mucus, which explains the 1.6 liters of fluid the thoracic surgeon drained from my right lung.
- **Sarcoma:** Sarcomas develop in connective tissue such as blood vessels, muscles, tendons, nerves, and bones. A carcinoma could develop a sarcoma after it has metastasized.
- **Leukemias and lymphomas:** These tumors develop in the glands or bone marrow. Lymphomas are designated as either Hodgkin lymphoma, meaning it involves the Reed-Sternberg cells, or the more

common non-Hodgkin lymphoma.

Cancer is also defined by its presentation and the rate at which it grows:

- **Well-differentiated tumors:** the tumor tissue resembles the surrounding tissue.
- **Undifferentiated tumors:** the tumor cells look different from the surrounding tissue and grow much faster than well-differentiated tumors.
- **High-grade cancer cells:** these fast and aggressive tumors typically have an extremely poor prognosis.

After hearing the word "incurable," many people would probably curl up, give in to depression, and pass away. But surrendering to cancer never felt like an option to me. If I had listened to my doctors and their statistics, I would not be here today.

My whole life, I had prioritized the needs of others over my own. Now, the time had come for me to put Veronica Villanueva first. I had dreams I wanted to fulfill, and more importantly, I had finally found my next purpose in life.

Mark Twain said, "The two most important days in your life are the day you are born and the day you find out why."

Cancer revealed my "why"—to help people discover their full potential, activate their inner strength, and heal from their struggles and pain as I healed from mine. In keeping with that mission, I intend to donate a portion of the proceeds from this book to a foundation that will help people with no means to afford naturopathic treatment. I am also looking to partner with integrative clinics that can donate their time and treatments so more people can have access to integrative medicine.

I'm here to prove to you that the impossible is possible. Most importantly, I want to show you the greatness and grace that exist in you and in everything around you. The world is full of beauty and wonder. It is time for you to open your eyes and see it, starting with you.

My healing journey taught me humility and revealed more blessings in my life than I could have imagined. I started out not knowing what to do or where to look for answers, but I learned the value of relinquishing my grip on things I cannot control and being open to possibilities. I prayed, "God, I am not asking you to take this cancer out of my body. I did this to myself, so I will get rid of it, but I need your help. I am asking you to guide me. Give me signs when I am going in the right direction and signs when I am on the wrong path, because I do not have much time. I promise to look for your signs, connect the dots, and stay open to anything that can heal me."

Sure enough, my prayers were answered. God and the universe guided me through my healing journey. I did not have an outline of steps to fight cancer, but I made sure to stay open-minded and feed my body and soul everything it needed to align with my decision to live. This included the tangible aspects of my healing journey—the treatments I did, the diet I ate, and the lifestyle changes I made—but also equally important, the spiritual and mental changes that freed me from stress and negativity.

YOUR CHEAT SHEET TO HEALING

"Tell the story of the mountain you climbed. Your words could become a page in someone else's survival guide."

—MORGAN HARPER NICHOLS

Fortunately, you *do* have an outline to healing: *this* book! I am alive today to share how my pain and struggles with cancer paved the way for my personal transformation— and how yours can do the same.

This book is the step-by-step guide on how I treated the cancer in my body using natural therapies and lifestyle as medicine. I discuss everything I learned and did in the first year and a half after the diagnosis. Cancer is a complex disease, and every day there are new findings that can help treat it. I am not claiming that I am cured of cancer, but I can celebrate having no tumors in my body. The same way I didn't listen to being labeled as having six months to live, I have learned that labeling where I am in my journey is not that important. The *most* important takeaway is that

I am thriving and feeling healthy, and my scans show no evidence of the disease.

The one *big* thing I would like to communicate to you, my reader, is the hope I believe we all must have despite the gloomy prognoses we are given. My faith and my belief brought me hope. Understand that physical, mental, and spiritual health are all connected, and they are all necessary ingredients to healing the disease in your body.

This book is a cheat sheet on how to treat your cancer. I had to figure out the steps on my own, but by using what I have learned, you will be able to take an accelerated path to the healthier, happier, best version of yourself. This path will save you precious time and money because you won't need to figure out what to do on your own—I'll ask the hard questions you might be afraid to ask your doctor *and* give you the answers so you can make lifesaving changes immediately.

You'll get the winning formula that rid my body of tumors, but you will also find tips you can follow the rest of your life to keep your illness from returning. Everyone can benefit from the lessons in these pages to live a full, healthy life unrestricted by stress and fear.

By following the lessons in this book, your body will gain homeostasis and holistically treat every aspect of your disease. You will choose what to eat and what thoughts to feed your mind. In turn, you can choose to stop poisoning your body with toxic, processed foods and to stop filling your head with negative thoughts. Once you learn to do this, you will begin to heal. You will thrive and find true, authentic happiness by letting go of the things you thought you could control. Instead, you will embrace the things you *can* control, like your lifestyle, diet, thoughts, and emotions.

Join me in the following chapters as we explore:

- What can cause cancer to develop in the body
- How a positive, growth-focused mindset is a major ingredient in your healing journey
- Why you need to believe in yourself to heal
- How the people around you can either support you or increase your stress
- Steps to educate yourself on your disease and treatment options
- The differences between Western and alternative medicine
- The role nutrition plays in healing
- Treatment options like cannabis, intravenous (IV) therapy, supplements, and more
- Lifestyle changes that will decrease and manage your stress and improve your overall health
- How to bring joy into your daily life

Your healing journey begins the minute you start believing in yourself. As a first step, you have a decision to make: how badly do you want to live?

I chose to believe in myself. I chose to open myself up to whatever signs and possibilities the universe sent my way. Above all, **I chose to live**—not a mediocre life but a phenomenal one!

My story is not unique—it could be your story, too. We are not victims of this disease, especially when we share our stories. I know that I would never want another person to feel the same way I did, and hopefully, by writing this book, I can reduce the stress of having this disease.

Cancer is not a death sentence, and together, we can change the conversation and add to the growing chorus of voices of people who lived. Let's replace cancer as a death sentence with cancer as a life sentence. It is a chance for you to create a healing environment where your body is nourished, your mind is limitless, you practice unstoppable belief, and you experience hope and joy on a daily basis.

You probably have a lot of questions—I did, too! I wrote this book to be the resource I wish I had when I was first diagnosed. Most books that exist today are theoretical and share the story of cancer diagnoses that were not labeled "incurable." Mine was stage 4 because it had metastasized, but it was also called incurable. As if being diagnosed with cancer is not depressing enough, being told that "your type of cancer is incurable" brings you to your knees.

This book does not need to be read in order. You can find the answers to the questions causing you the most anxiety before flipping back to learn more. Like ordering from a menu, I want you to pick and choose the advice that applies the most to you.

You have the power to heal if you are willing to believe in yourself and join me as we explore the path to a healthier, holistic lifestyle.

As Lance Armstrong said, "We have two options, medically and emotionally: give up or fight like hell."

What will you decide?

Chapter 1

THE DECISION TO LIVE

THE WORLD IS BETTER WITH ME IN IT

"You become what you think about."

—NAPOLEON HILL

You have a **choice**: live or die. Which one will it be?

I hope by reading my story, you will choose the obvious, TO LIVE!

This chapter is all about putting yourself in the right mindset to begin your healing journey. I will share the story of receiving my diagnosis and how I refused to "give up," and I will explain why you, too, need to make a conscious decision to be brave and fight. Making that decision means focusing on the outcome you want for yourself, removing negativity from your life, and being open to trying anything that will help you heal. I'll also explore the difference between choosing to *survive* and choosing to *live*, and why you need to do the latter. It's not enough to be on autopilot; you need to be alive and engaged in life to thrive.

THE START OF HEALING: MY STORY

"The courage it takes to share your story might be the very thing someone else needs to open their heart to hope."

—UNKNOWN

The day of my diagnosis, it took me an hour to roll out of bed because I was in so much pain. I could not get up vertically because I had such a hard time breathing. I lay in bed and had to strategize how to stand. The only way was to roll to my side and use my elbow to push myself up. Next, I struggled to dress myself in my workout clothes to feel somewhat comfortable. I kept thinking, *hurry up*, because I was afraid I would stop breathing.

Luckily, when I arrived at the hospital at four in the morning, practically crawling into the emergency room, unable to breathe, the admitting nurse rushed me into my own room. My wonderful female doctor quickly ordered all kinds of tests while professionals rushed in and out of my room to draw blood and perform ultrasounds. The doctor scanned my body and told me I looked too healthy to have anything seriously wrong with me. She was sure that whatever I had was just the flu.

The next time I saw that doctor, she leaned over, hugged me, and said, "Sweetie, you have cancer." She went on to explain that I had 1.6 liters of fluid in my right lung. The fluid was caused by the cancer, which is why I felt pain in my back.

If I could not breathe beforehand, hearing that news took away all the breath I had left. I could barely utter any words, and I was in so much shock that I could not even cry. A line of doctors waited outside my room: the pulmonologist, cardiothoracic surgeon, oncologist, and others. Everyone seemed perplexed. On paper, I looked healthy. All my blood work came back fine, except for the cancer.

There was a big debate about whether I should have surgery that day. On the one hand, I needed surgery as soon as possible; if left untreated, the immense pressure from the 1.6 liters of fluid in my right lung could resolve and collapse. The pulmonologists asked me when my back pain started and when I first felt fatigued. It was a surreal experience to be asked questions I was nowhere near prepared to answer. The doctors finally agreed that I needed surgery as soon as possible.

I arrived at the emergency room on Thursday, September 22, 2016. By that Saturday, I had surgery to drain the fluid from my right lung. I wanted to wait for my daughters, Mirabella and Karina, to make it to the hospital before my surgery. One lived in New York and the other was at Stanford.

For the thoracic surgery, I had two incisions below my right breast. The doctors inserted a tube to drain the fluid from my lung. Today, I look at the two scars as my battle scars that remind me that cancer tried to weaken my courage, take over my soul, and destroy my hope. I am stronger than this disease. During the surgery, they removed 1600mL of fluids from my right pleural space, which they biopsied.

When I woke up from surgery, I remember seeing my two beautiful daughters. I did—and do—love them more than anything. I could not bear the thought of never seeing them again. Even without the results of the biopsy, the doctor had already confirmed that I had cancer, based on his extensive experience. While I was still sleeping from the anesthesia, he told my daughters I would not qualify for chemotherapy nor radiation. My pathology report reads: "Metastatic non-cell adenocarcinoma of the lung on a pleural biopsy. The malignant cells were TTF-1 positive."

The doctors listed and described the tumors I had on the left side, which had spread to my pelvis and upper abdominal area. On the right side, my tumors were labeled as extensive, stretching from my right armpit all the way down the right side of my body.

Despite already experiencing symptoms in February 2016, I chose to ignore the signs. Even my acupuncturist said that the pain was coming from my right lung and advised me to get it checked by a doctor. That was the first sign I ignored. My best friend from San Francisco also told me to see a doctor, but I said I had no time and probably hurt myself playing tennis.

Frankly, my wellbeing was not a priority back then. If it did not fit with my schedule, it was not important.

WHAT DOES IT MEAN TO BE HEALTHY?

"The mind and the body are not separate. What affects one, affects the other."

—ANONYMOUS

In all honesty, at that point in my life, I felt invincible. Obviously, I had heard horror stories about other people getting ill, but I never thought something like that would happen to me.

The problem was that I never fully understood what being healthy meant. My misguided ticket to never being sick was over-exercising and eating right. I ate fairly well and cooked five days a week. I did not drink or do drugs like so many other people. How could *I* be sick?

Clearly, I had missed the connection between the mind and body. The way you live your life and the thoughts you think have a huge impact on your internal health, which I never realized. By living in a stressful and unhappy state for so many years, I had created a disease in my body. Although I did the right things for my physical appearance, I was damaging myself internally.

Before my diagnosis, I had an exciting plan for the next chapter of my life. I was forty-nine years old, but I felt half my age. I was full of confidence, ready to make a name for myself. My children were independent, and my marriage had finally ended. In 2016, I was supposed to live the high life in Los Angeles. I dreamt of becoming an entrepreneur and being a healthy cultured chef, traveling all over the world to learn cooking from different countries. When I returned to the United States, I would expose people to other cultures of the world through food.

The year I was diagnosed with cancer taught me a real lesson in humility. The first step to healing was to accept that I had cancer. I, Veronica Villanueva, had a disease despite believing I had a bulletproof body. The disease quickly started eating my muscle away, leaving me looking frail. I dropped to eighty-nine pounds with a BMI of 18.1. I no longer resembled my old self. Not physically, anyway.

Quickly, I was forced to detach myself from the life I had planned and the person I was. At that point, I was not in control—God was.

LIFE OR DEATH?

"See, I have set before you this day, life and good, death and evil...I have set before you life and death, blessing and curse, therefore choose life."

—MOSES, DEUTERONOMY 30:15-19

During my first real conversation with my oncologist, he explained that I had stage 4 metastatic lung cancer. I learned that stage 4 meant the disease had spread to several areas in my body, which is why I could not do chemotherapy or radiation. My entire upper body was a target.

"Let's cure it then," I said.

"There is no cure," he replied. That is when he told me I had six months to live.

Luckily, I believed the world was a better place *with* me than without me. I was **not going anywhere.** You should have seen his facial expression. Well-intentioned, his face showed deep concern and sadness because he felt sorry for me. Clearly, I was not accepting the diagnosis I had been given. According to him, he was dealing with a patient in denial. *No*, he was dealing with a badass warrior who refused to succumb to this horrific and painful disease!

When you are diagnosed with cancer, your Western oncologist will either recommend surgery, radiation, chemotherapy, or a combination of multiple treatments. The modern approach to cancer is "slash, burn, and poison."[1] In retrospect, it was a blessing to be spared the pressure of having to make this decision. Although traditional chemotherapy and radiation are appropriate for certain types of cancer, I am glad my case was not one of them.

I had to look for an alternative way to heal: natural and holistic. This meant breaking and replacing bad habits. When I received my diagnosis, I had reached a dead-end in Western medicine. As far as the doctors were concerned, there was nothing they could do for me. It was just a matter of time before I died!

Naturally, I started searching for someone to give me more hope. While I knew that diet and proper nutrition were important to good health, *that* alone would not reverse the disease. To get rid of the tumors that plagued my upper body, I knew I had to do things that I had never done before. I had to do something drastic to rebuild my internal terrain.

Integrative medicine, which I'll explore in detail later in the book, changed my life. I began asking the right questions to help me better understand the cancer in my body.

---

1 Winters, Nasha, and Jess Higgins Kelley. *The Metabolic Approach to Cancer: Integrating Deep Nutrition, the Ketogenic Diet, and Nontoxic Bio-Individualized Therapies.* White River Junction, VT: Chelsea Green Publishing, 2017.

I uncovered the root cause of the disease by exploring all the modalities to heal my body. Most importantly, I learned the steps required to start healing. For the first time, **I was given hope**. Nobody was telling me I was going to die anymore.

Every Western doctor I spoke to apologized for not being able to help me. I did not want anyone feeling sorry for me, which is why integrative medicine felt so refreshing. Suddenly, I had options other than dying!

PREPARING TO CLIMB THE MOUNTAIN

"When your desires are strong enough, you will appear to possess superhuman powers to achieve."

—NAPOLEON HILL

Healing starts in your mind. First, you need to visualize the life you want to live. This vision becomes your new reality.

Deciding your outcome is by far the hardest thing to do in life—for everyone, but especially when you have been diagnosed with a serious illness. Our goals and dreams often feel impossibly far away, as though they sit on the peak of a high mountain. When we look up at the summit and think about reaching those goals, we feel discouraged and overwhelmed before we even take our first step.

After learning my diagnosis, being so close to mortality magnified my focus on the outcome I wanted: **to live**. Yes, it was hard for me to see this at first, and it will be hard for you, too. You are given an overwhelming amount of information from your doctors. Look past the distractions, decide and commit to your new life, and, finally, visualize it.

Choosing to live feels like aiming for the top of the mountain, but you *will* reach it if you take the steps and commit to the process. I am living proof that what you think is impossible is, in fact, *possible.*

When I first heard my diagnosis, I told myself, "Veronica, look up once. Remember the top of the mountain, but don't look up again. Just take a step forward every day." The same goes for breathing and walking again—one baby step that required so much effort from my lungs. I will never take breathing for granted again.

Think about it, what downsides are there to deciding to live? NONE! I was already given a death sentence, so I believed I could only win from that point on. If anything, this death sentence has pushed me even more to live a meaningful and fulfilled life!

Nine months later, I reached the top of the mountain when I received my first clean scan. Today, I say cancer is the best thing that ever happened to me because everything I learned and discovered during the healing process paved the way for my new life of fulfillment.

None of the beautiful experiences I've had since my diagnosis would have happened if I hadn't decided to live. The first step to making that decision for yourself is knowing what you want to live *for*. What do you want out of life? By asking this compelling question, it brings awareness that your thoughts and efforts determine your behavior and actions.

Visualize the life you want for yourself. What are you fighting for? Is it something miserable or extraordinary?

I knew what I wanted as my outcome: to get rid of the cancer in my body and live a healthier and happier life than before. Once you have clarity on the direction you will take, it is time to make your path easier to travel by removing the negativity from your life.

IDENTIFY THE SOURCES OF NEGATIVITY IN YOUR LIFE

"Only those who can see the invisible, can do the impossible."

—FRANK GAINES

When I got sick, I realized I had experienced years of chronic negative emotions like sadness, anxiety, and loneliness, all of which contributed to the illness.

My family life looked perfect from the outside, but little did everyone know, inside I experienced emotional chaos—a storm brewing, a *disease* brewing. I smiled to the world while weeping inside. I lived in an unhappy marriage and suffered from intense loneliness and guilt for not being happy when everyone in my social circle thought I had everything a woman could want: a successful husband, three beautiful children, a large home, and trips around the world.

Yes, *why* would I not be happy in my marriage?

Now I know the reason for my misery. I tried to control every aspect of my life because I wanted my children to see me as the perfect Super Mom I never had growing up. I also desperately wanted to protect them. Instead of realizing that certain things were out of my control, like what my children did when I was not around to watch them, I worried constantly and kept my emotions bottled inside me like poison.

My anxiety worsened as my children aged. I remember the moment I became a chronically anxious mother. When my daughter was young, she split open her lip. Blood poured everywhere, and as I rushed her to the emergency room, I realized, *Oh my god. She can be taken away from me.* I lost my own father in a plane crash when I was not even seven years old, so I think I internalized the fear of losing a loved one more than most people. I mistook the anxiety and fight-or-flight rush I felt in the traumatic situation with my daughter for strength, without realizing how much the negative emotions hurt my body and mind. Over the following years, I never found a healthier way to process my concern and worries for my children.

At the same time, I obsessed over my tennis playing and busy social life. I thought by staying occupied and surrounding myself with friends, I could mask the pain of my aching heart, which so desperately craved the intimacy lacking in my marriage.

I began going through divorce proceedings shortly before my diagnosis. I knew I needed to make changes in my life to be happy and had started to make plans. I wanted to travel, work as a chef, date, and, for once, put myself first. I had *so many* reasons to live, and now my doctor was telling me I wouldn't get the chance to do any of it? I thought *no way!*

I decided to live a life full of love, adventure, and service to others—*that* would be my outcome. But I also realized I couldn't control exactly how I reached that destination and I couldn't plan out every detail of my recovery. To some extent, I had already learned this lesson from my failed marriage and my children: you can't control everything, and when you try, things often don't go as planned.

Before the cancer diagnosis, I wanted to control every aspect of my life, to the extent that when I left my children with a babysitter, I would write out a minute-by-minute agenda. *From one to two o'clock, sit in front of the window and have my babies look at the trees while listening to Mozart in preparation for their naps.*

I tried so hard to be the perfect Super Mom, but attempting to manage the aspects of my life that were out of my control only caused anxiety, which undoubtedly contributed to the cancer in my body. All that negativity and unhappiness built up and affected me psychologically and physiologically for years.

I believe the unhappiness and negativity primed my body for disease and set the wheels in motion, but the shock of my divorce is what ultimately triggered the cancer. I had expected to have an amicable divorce with my husband, and because I went into the separation in good faith, I believed he had done the same. In hindsight, it was naïve of me to believe he would treat me with the same respect I had given him.

Little did I know he had been collecting years of "evidence" to paint me in a poor light. He compiled documents, emails, and text messages behind my back in an attempt to win a favorable outcome in the divorce proceedings, all while leading me to believe we could divorce amicably. When I realized he had built an extensive case against me while I had nothing to defend myself with, the shock was unbelievable. I remember thinking about the position I was in and saying to myself, "I'm doomed," and I believe *that* was the moment that triggered the cancer. The mind and body share a powerful connection, and by speaking those words, I had told my body that my life was *over*.

By the time I received my diagnosis, I knew I had to stop worrying and open myself up to whatever possibilities the universe and God brought my way. For the first time in my life, I had to be okay with not knowing what would happen next and learn to be happy despite the prognosis I was given.

I want you to look at your life. What is making you unhappy or causing you stress? My anxiety and desire to control every aspect of my life were huge sources of negativity and unhappiness, and I think a lot of people struggle to let go of control. However, you need to accept that you cannot control everything as you face your illness and open yourself up to anything that can help you live.

Your life will need to change, and what is important is that you *keep living a fulfilling life*.

HOPE CALLS FOR ACTION: A LIMITLESS MINDSET

"Never, never, never give up."

—WINSTON CHURCHILL

I didn't only want to *survive* and overcome the cancer; I wanted to live an extraordinary life!

Choosing to live also meant choosing to live a *different* life. I would be starting from a blank canvas, but I knew if I stayed confident and truly believed in my goal to live a beautiful and fulfilling life, I would be graced with the signs I needed to move in the right direction.

Any one of us can set an intention to live. But an intention is not enough. Never underestimate the power of commitment and discipline when building your dream life.

The decision to live comes from identifying *your* asset. What can you do?

For example, one of my greatest assets was, and still is, studying. I exposed myself to so many books in the early days after my diagnosis. My days were spent reading and researching. The more I studied, the less I felt like I was going crazy. I found stories of people who had recovered from cancer. I realized my decision to live was possible *if* I put myself in a positive mindset and committed to living *right now*, not in the past as that would only make me depressed. I needed to live in the present, which would reward me with the feeling of gratitude.

In other words, when you choose to live, you have to *continue* to live. This means not staying home all the time; you need to leave your house and get out in the world. Aside from the fact that I lost weight, I never looked sick because I believed by looking sick, I would stay sick. I continued to function and be part of the world. I refused to be depressed and stay in bed. I surrounded myself with loving friends and laughed on a daily basis. Sometimes, this meant adjusting my lifestyle to accommodate for the illness. For example, I cut sugar and animal products from my diet. If I went out to a restaurant with friends, I either ordered steamed vegetables or ate before. By making these changes, I was able to continue to live my life and not put it on hold because of cancer. I told my friends to be as normal as possible around me because I did not want any pity. They drank wine while I sipped on my hot water with lemon or mint tea. Nobody treated me like a victim, which was important to me.

Every day, you have to show that you are living your life to the fullest. Your body will respond to that effort. When I made the decision to live, I also chose not to isolate myself. I deliberately did *not* want to live a sick life. If you live a sick life, your body will follow.

Remember, the key is to prime your mind for healing. If you continue living, you will live. If you continue to live in a sick way, you will be sick.

One of my client's wives was diagnosed with breast cancer. The couple always lived a glamorous life. My client opened up to me about how he constantly encouraged his wife to go out and eat dinner with their friends, but all she wanted was to stay home. She lost her hair, so she did not feel pretty enough to see people. In my opinion, this is a dangerous approach that will cause your mental and physical health to suffer.

Instead, I want you to not only strive for a normal life but aim to make every day *extraordinary*. When you decide to fight to live, honor your choice by doing everything in your power to make your life exciting. **Survival is not a good enough goal.**

We are all guilty of taking life too seriously. Adults forget to live like kids, but no matter what they do, kids always have a great time. I have learned a lot about life from observing the way children behave. They move through the world free of anxiety and other negative emotions.

When you choose to live, make sure you are living a life worth fighting for. If anything feels gloomy and unfulfilling, change it. This is your chance to redesign your life.

Deciding to live is the first step. The next step is to ask yourself what *kind* of life you want to live. Know what you want to work towards.

Isolating yourself from the rest of the world to be miserable at home is not living. When you choose to live, you choose to make life exciting. *That* is your medicine. The consequence of living an exciting life is effectively curing yourself.

It can be difficult to continue living when your illness causes symptoms like pain or nausea—sensations that will distract you, hurt your morale, and hold you back from the activities you enjoy—but you can take steps to mentally fortify yourself against the discomfort.

MIND OVER MATTER: FEEL "NO" PAIN

"At the subatomic level, energy responds to your mindful attention and becomes matter."

—DR. JOE DISPENZA

In February 2016, I experienced intense back pain, so I went to an acupuncturist. I frequently played tennis, so I thought my backhand had inflamed or pulled a muscle in my back. My acupuncturist, however, told me to have my doctor examine it. Apparently, my back was not the problem, but my lung. I ignored her advice and didn't visit a doctor.

During this time, I rarely spoke to my friends and family about my discomfort. As always, I wanted to be Super Mom. If I did not talk about my pain, maybe it would cease to exist.

Fast forward to June of that year, when I caught the flu and never fully recovered. From that point, I started growing weaker and weaker. Finally, I was diagnosed in September 2016 with lung cancer, seven months after the initial back pain had started.

It turns out that part of having lung cancer is the pain on your back. I also had pain in my pelvis and stomach. I remember thinking to myself that, if I wanted my pain to go away, I should stop complaining about it. I suspected I could combat the pain by putting myself in the right mindset, but my doctor prescribed morphine and other painkillers.

I did not take a single painkiller medication.

I had a gut feeling that medicine would do nothing good for me. Only after my research did I learn how dangerous medicine can be and how many toxins it can release into your body.

My mind served as my strongest coping strategy. I knew that focusing on the pain would only make it hurt more. It's one thing to acknowledge the pain but to accept it is something I was not prepared to do. As Friedrich Nietzsche once said, "He who has a 'why' to live can bear almost any how. To live is to suffer, to survive is to find some meaning in the suffering. That which does not kill us makes us stronger."

Instead, I told myself, "Nothing hurts. I feel great." I repeated this message to myself over and over until, one day, it was true! I no longer felt any pain.

It took time to reach this point where I could shut out my discomfort, and I would be lying if I said lung cancer was not painful. Lung cancer is *very* painful; my back and abdomen hurt a *lot*. One time, in January 2017, I was in so much pain that I was hospitalized. As I lay in the hospital bed, I told myself, "Veronica, this is the last time you will feel this sort of pain." And it was. Since then, I have never felt pain like I did in that moment.

Just like you can decide to live, you can decide how much power you will give to your pain. Focus on taking away your pain's strength, and you can fight through it. You can continue to live your life to the fullest without giving up the activities you enjoy. Over time, if you mentally resist your pain and shift your focus, you will feel it less and less.

As you start your healing journey, you might find that your loved ones don't always support your decisions. For example, they might insist you take painkillers or stay home to rest when you want to do the opposite.

You know your body and your own capabilities better than anyone else, so this is the next step in deciding to live: you need to live for yourself.

CHOOSE TO LIVE FOR YOURSELF

"If you want to achieve greatness, stop asking for permission."

—UNKNOWN

In deciding to live, you need to both make the choice *by yourself* and *for yourself.*

When faced with a diagnosis, it is important to talk to your family. Make sure they understand your situation and let them know you love them. Ultimately, however, you need to put yourself first. You become your own advocate. The best thing anyone else can do is to be 100 percent supportive of you, but often, people will want to make choices on your behalf.

Thinking about other people, especially the people closest to us, complicates our decision-making process when we are navigating an illness. If someone challenges your decisions or tries to pressure you into something that makes you uncomfortable, remind yourself that

your diagnosis is about you first and fore
nobody else.

Ideally, your family and friends will posit
the same page as you. To avoid judgme
your decision-making process easier, surround yourself
with people who can respect and align themselves with
your choices. Anybody who lacks alignment should not be
part of your new world, at least not for the first few months
of your healing journey.

In exceptionally difficult circumstances, the last thing you
want is to create extra hurdles for yourself. When so much
is out of your control, remember that you can control who
you choose to have around you and how they help *you* in
your decision.

As humans, our default is to think negatively. We constantly doubt ourselves, which is especially challenging
when you first receive a diagnosis. It can be tempting
to defer to the people around you and allow them to
make your decisions, but don't give up your power and
autonomy. Making your own decisions will empower you
to continue living and replace your negative thoughts
with more positive ones. You will gain enough courage
to distance yourself from people who make it difficult
to stay committed to your decisions, and instead put
yourself first.

some weird reason, whenever we take time to take care of ourselves, we feel selfish and guilty. Self-care is *not* selfish, and especially not when you are sick. Taking care of yourself means listening to what your body and mind are telling you. Do not feel guilty for this.

First, take the time to be still. You have to turn down—or even turn off—the volume of your surroundings. Being still is being courageous. It is during this silence that you will open yourself up to receiving the grace of God and or the universe's guidance. Both are fighting the battle for you. **Believe!**

When I was in labor with one of my children, all I wanted to hear was my doctor's voice and my ex-husband showing me how to breathe. At that moment, nothing else mattered. I did not want to acknowledge any other noise, because it did not contribute to me feeling calm. By choosing to focus on what was helping me, I tuned everything else out. My goal was to get my baby out as soon as possible and be focused while doing so.

You need to find the same personal focus. For once in your life, sit with *yourself*. When you listen to your body and mind, you allow for something magical to happen. This could be religious, like a message from God, or spiritual, like a sign from the universe.

With silence comes clarity and freedom. Any noise around

you can distract from your own decisions. When you cannot hear yourself think, you cannot possibly know what you want. In moments of solitude, decisions will find their way to you. The only way to make a goal happen is to own it yourself. *You* have to make that happen. Not your husband, not your children. YOU!

This is *your* decision to live. Putting other people's needs ahead of your own will not sustain you throughout this difficult journey. You need to draw from inner strength and put yourself first, and you cannot do that if you do not love yourself.

LEARN TO LOVE YOURSELF UNAPOLOGETICALLY

"To be yourself in a world that is constantly trying to make you something else is the greatest accomplishment."

—RALPH WALDO EMERSON

If you do not love yourself, what do you have to live for? To truly be happy and healthy, you need to make the decision to live by yourself and for yourself. **When you express self-love, you say no to dying and yes to living.**

Part of loving yourself is embracing your purpose and creating a mission for yourself. When you decide to live, you need to understand *why*. What makes you feel fulfilled in life? You need to redefine or find that meaning for yourself.

Consider your reasons for wanting to live. How many of those reasons are about other people? How many are about you?

Personally, I wanted to live because I had so many plans for myself. For once, I did not include my children in my decision. Instead, I prioritized my freedom. I wanted to live according to what *I* thought *my* life could be. I was desperate for an authenticity I always felt I lacked in the past.

Your life is yours for a reason. You should not be living for other people. You are living because you matter; your children are living because they matter.

Unfortunately, women have been put in a difficult position over the centuries. We feel a lot of guilt about who we are supposed to be as women, mothers, and wives. This guilt shaped my unhappiness. I did things I thought I was supposed to do, instead of those I actually wanted to do. After my diagnosis, it was time to live the life that *I* wanted.

If you feel guilt, it is time to forgive yourself. Forgiveness means freeing yourself from all the negative feelings inside of you, including resentment or regret. When you forgive yourself, you let go of whatever happened in the past and accept that you did your best. At the end of the day, that is what we are all trying to do: our best. *That* should be enough.

There is no sense in punishing yourself. You should not punish yourself for being sick, for example. Instead, see this as an opportunity or a lesson. See and understand the purpose of the pain you are feeling. Recognizing that you have the right to choose to live is an expression of self-love. This means you love yourself so much that you believe the world is better with you in it. As a human being, you have something to contribute to the world.

Making this decision to live and love yourself is your opportunity to exercise your authority and take back control. Your decision matters, just like your life matters.

This is your time to make yourself a priority, and nobody can fault you for it. Stand up for yourself first. Chances are people will judge you no matter what treatment you choose—tune them out. In my case, my doctor dismissed my decision to stop eating sugar. He said there was never anything wrong with my diet. I had always been healthy, which is why everyone was so surprised I had cancer.

Instead of fighting my doctor on that point, I chose to ignore him. I had enough to focus on without arguing about my diet. My energy went towards healing myself and beating the cancer inside me. It was pointless to justify what I was doing to anyone. For once in my life, my dignified silence was the answer. Silence and patience are necessary to heal.

Like everything else I put my mind to, I became a master of taking care of myself. I knew I was good at it as I had given that same effort to my children and my ex-husband. Never towards myself, sadly, until that point. After my diagnosis, I put all my energy toward healing my body, and if anyone or anything was taxing my energy in a detrimental way, I chose to ignore it. Remember, you can choose which people are around you. The last thing you need is unnecessary drama.

Throughout this process, you might feel very alone. The people around you might not understand your decisions or your actions. They might pass judgment or offer advice of their own. You do not have to justify or explain your decisions. It's *your* life! Trust yourself. Remember, this is not about your husband, your kids, or your friends. *Your* process should be right for *you*. At the end of the day, this is all that matters.

Gaining control of your life is a cumulative process. The first step is to make the decision to live. When you make that decision, you sign up to do the work required to live your dream life. Part of choosing to live is deciding deliberately to avoid anything that will steer you away from your positive mindset.

POSITIVITY IS KEY TO HEALING

"We are twice armed if we fight with faith."

—PLATO

Your body reacts to the thoughts you feed it, and the only way to heal is to start this journey with a positive mindset. Every word that comes out of your mouth, every thought that enters your mind, everything you do, and everything you eat has to align with your healing. There are *no* exceptions!

There is no way to trick your body or take shortcuts. Understand that your diet is not just about what you eat. It's the people that you surround yourself with, what you listen to, and what you read and watch. In order for healing to be possible, you have to stay consistent. You must believe in the powerful connection between your mind, body, and soul.

When we hear the word "cancer," we often jump straight to death. That is the default for most people, but it does not have to be. You can change your default associations and assumptions. In fact, you have to if you want to heal.

The bottom line is that you have two options: you can die, or you can live.

Naturally, you will experience negative thoughts, especially when you receive your diagnosis. You are human after all. However, it is all about the mindset. When you decide to live, you commit to taking *positive* actions, which means you cannot continue with those same disempowering thoughts. This does not mean ignoring them when they arise. Instead, you can acknowledge your negative thoughts and replace them with an empowering set of emotions. Your thoughts, your perceptions, your emotions, and your reactions are all within your control. The truth is this: positivity is all up to you!

I dealt with a lot of my negative thoughts by educating myself. Information should empower you and propel you forward. The more you see and understand the ways in which you are healing yourself, the more you will embrace the concept as a whole.

In the same way you go to the gym to strengthen your muscles, you must work hard to reinforce your positive mindset. In the first week of working out, you probably will not notice much definition in your body. However, if you stay consistent and disciplined, you might start to notice your biceps toning up. You will start to feel stronger.

The little things you add into your days and weeks become cumulative. The more you practice positivity, the more you can build your muscle of hope, mental strength, and agility.

You cannot reverse a disease without first reversing the way you think. This process starts with mindfulness and being aware of your thoughts—do not let negativity run rampant through your mind! As I mentioned earlier, our automatic default is to think negatively. Every time you catch yourself thinking negatively, you have an opportunity to reverse that thinking. You can rewire your mind to think good thoughts. Start by *feeling* gratitude. You are still alive, after all.

You can learn to shift your thoughts from negative to positive like any other skill, but it takes practice, being mindful, and living in the moment. It takes recognizing the words that are coming out of your mouth and the thoughts crossing through your head.

Remember, your goal should not be to survive. Your goal should be to *LIVE!* When you adopt a positive mindset, you are actively choosing to live a phenomenal life.

When I made the decision to live, I wanted to be healthier than I was before my diagnosis. My past mistakes and negativity were no longer part of my formula. When *you* choose to live, you must be open to transformation and everything it entails. Your old way of living led to sickness, so now it is time to change directions.

WHY?

"Greatness does not come from trying to achieve the possible."

—CONSTANCE FRIDAY

As you continue along your healing journey, remind yourself of your *why*. Hold on to the image you created of your dream outcome—the top of your mountain.

Think of it in the same way you might picture your "goal body" when you start going to the gym. You might imagine it, or even print out a photo and hang it on your wall for motivation. On easy days, you might not even look at the picture because your goal is already in your head. On days where you feel like quitting, you can refer to the image and remind yourself *why* you are working out in the first place.

Picture the life you want to live and refer to that image daily.

Personally, I have always loved the beach, heat, and sun. When I decided to live, I envisioned myself living on the beach and looking out over the ocean every day. Now, that is exactly what I am doing. I knew I wanted nature to be a big part of my daily life. I made my dream a reality because I believed in myself and manifested my goals.

Now that you have made your decision, **to live**, it is time to believe in it.

JOURNAL EXERCISE: WRITING YOUR EULOGY

As I processed my diagnosis and began my healing journey, I learned that journaling can be a powerful tool for channeling emotions and detoxing your mind. Instead of dwelling on negative thoughts, I wrote them down. I wrote about everything, from not liking my landlord to not having enough time to research new therapies. After a few months of journaling, I noticed patterns in my writing. I also realized I had fewer and fewer negative things to write about. By getting the thoughts out of my head, I was able to process them and move on.

I recommend starting a journal now and documenting your experience. Make journaling a part of your morning ritual so you can set up your day for success.

As you continue through this book, I will guide you in thought exercises that will help you transform your mind and life, starting with this one: writing your eulogy.

Writing your eulogy is an opportunity to consider how you are affecting other people. When faced with your mortality, you naturally start to wonder what people will say about you when you pass away.

Not only did I think about what others would say about me, but what I would say about *myself*. So, I wrote my own eulogy.

When I read my eulogy to my friends, they made me feel good about what I had written. I was the person they went to for health advice because they trusted my opinion. Not only did I make them laugh, but I inspired them too. In the early days after my diagnosis, I found great comfort and motivation in knowing I had a positive impact on the people around me.

It might sound crazy, but writing your own eulogy is a great way to check in with yourself. It can help you compare how you wish to be remembered with the way you are currently living and solidify why, exactly, you want to live.

How would you like to be remembered? Remember, every day is a chance to transform your life and the way you live it. If there is something missing, identify it and write it in your journal.

Once you know the effect you want to have on the world, you can make the necessary changes to shape your dream life.

As an example, here is the eulogy I wrote for myself:

I have a beautiful mind, and I'm always ready to have deep conversations about you and life. I consider this to be one of my sacred moments.

The older I get, the more I crave one-on-one quality time with the people I love.

I love learning about anything that will make me a better person.

I love going out but prefer to cuddle and stay home with someone I love.

What makes me smile? Cooking for my loved ones and eating together while sharing stories.

My outer shell is tough and strong, but my inner soul is soft and, at times, fragile.

I am such a giver in every way. I love giving and recently learned to appreciate receiving.

You can get me to do anything for you when you smile

and put your arms around me.

I am naïve because I believe everyone in the world is good and no one is out to hurt me, despite being blindly hurt by my husband.

I love living a life that is filled with spontaneity and fun.

I go after what I want.

I am a true romantic. My essence is LOVE.

Chapter 2

BELIEF

EMBRACE THE POWER OF YOUR MIND

"Believe you can and you're halfway there."

—THEODORE ROOSEVELT

You can only make your decision to live a reality if you *believe* in your choice and in yourself. It is not enough to say the words, "I am going to live." You need to own them.

I would not be alive today if I had not believed in myself. I believed in my ability to overcome the disease in my body even when other people did not. My doctor declared the cancer "incurable," and my daughters told me it was okay to give up because they didn't want me to struggle and be in pain. But I believed in myself and knew I had the strength to fight back—to not only *survive*, but to live and become the person I am supposed to be! Cancer would not take me away from this beautiful world that I was so excited to be a part of.

The life and dreams I envisioned for myself were worth the struggle, and they only came true because I believed they would. I have this belief deeply, unshakably ingrained in my body, and I want you to feel the same.

There are four types of belief you need to adopt as you start your healing journey: you must believe in yourself, believe in a higher power that wants you to succeed, believe in your treatments, and believe in the people advising you. Each type of belief will play a key role in your recovery by reinforcing your positive mindset.

BELIEVE IN YOURSELF

"But, all things considered, it is possible for one man to do something that another man has achieved."

—TARUN BETALA

In the early days after the cancer diagnosis, my greatest moment of enlightenment happened when I recognized the immense power of the mind. My thoughts didn't exist outside of my body; they directly influenced my physical health. In fact, the first two steps in my healing journey, deciding to live and then believing in myself, both took place in my mind. The mind and body share a deep connection, and I realized my body could not be healthy unless I fed my mind empowering thoughts.

Your thoughts *hurt* you when you experience stress or think negatively, and they *heal* you when you think positively and love yourself. This ability to influence the body makes the mind an amazingly effective healing tool you can use to overcome your illness. To harness the power of your mind, you first need to believe in yourself.

TAKE RESPONSIBILITY

"Most people do not really want freedom, because freedom involves responsibility, and most people are frightened of responsibility."

—SIGMUND FREUD

I am not the product of my circumstances. I am the product of my decision—TO LIVE! A key part of believing in yourself is believing you have the power to change your circumstances. When I first heard my diagnosis, I knew I did not deserve to be sick, but I also realized I had harmed myself by allowing negativity, emotional pain, and stress into my life. I had to take responsibility for my health.

By owning everything from the negative thoughts and pressure I put on myself to the foods I ate and the lifestyle I lived, I empowered myself. If I had the power to damage my body, then I had the power to reverse it. I believed in my ability to change my mindset, behavior, habits, and health to achieve a remarkable life, and now I'm living it!

OVERCOME YOUR MENTAL DEFAULTS

"When someone tells me no, it doesn't mean I can't do it, it simply means I can't do it with them."

—KAREN E. QUINONES MILLER

"Believe in yourself" is often easier said than done, especially when facing a cancer diagnosis. When we first hear a poor prognosis, the default option is to believe in death, not in yourself. You must overcome this mental default because your thoughts influence your body, which makes defaulting to death like ingesting poison. In other words, you will not heal if you do not believe it is possible.

I've seen firsthand the benefits of believing in yourself, and I want you to see them, too. You might struggle with belief at first because we have been programmed from childhood to have what I call a "mental weakness default." Our default is to assume the worst; to think *I'm going to die* when we hear we are sick, regardless of the prognosis. But once you get past that default and start believing in your capacity to do the "impossible," the positive outcomes that naturally follow will reinforce your belief. This becomes your new mindset: believing that there is no storm so big that you can't weather it. Over time, believing in yourself and in your positive outcome will become your new default. You'll see the empowerment and change that comes from belief and say, "Oh my God, this is really working." After that, your belief will be untouchable.

DON'T LET STRUGGLES SHAKE YOUR BELIEF

"You can make plans, but the Lord's purpose will prevail."

—PROVERBS 19:21

Life is filled with struggles. Embrace them because discomfort is part of growth. As soon as you recognize these challenges as an opportunity to grow, they will not be able to shake your belief. When I received my diagnosis, I knew it was not a question of God or the universe punishing me. There was a reason I got sick, which meant there was a lesson to be learned. I had the opportunity to transform my diagnosis into something positive. This is what it means to be in charge of your mind.

Do not ask for your pain and struggles to go away; pray that you become stronger instead. There is always beauty to be found in your pain, and if you believe a positive side exists to your struggles, transformation is inevitable.

BELIEVE IN A HIGHER POWER

"When we stop trying to control events, they fall into a natural order, an order that works. We're at rest while a power much greater than our own takes over, and it does a much better job than we could have done. We learn to trust that the power that holds galaxies together can handle the circumstances of our relatively little lives."

—MARIANNE WILLIAMSON

Not only should you believe in a higher power, but you should believe that there is something out there to help and guide you. God never gives you anything you cannot handle, and nobody is out to punish you, either. It is a gift and privilege to be given a chance to grow. Surrender! As children, we expect to grow and change, but when we become adults, many people think the process stops. They fight change when they should instead surrender to it. To grow and improve, you need to open yourself up to change.

Any pain we experience is self-inflicted. Pain is a sign that you are living in an imbalanced way. For example, imagine you are in a toxic relationship. The universe did not force you to be with that person. Chances are you made excuses to stay in the relationship despite its negativity. When you feel emotional or physical pain, your body and mind are telling you something in your life needs to change.

By choosing to live in a positive and expansive way, you

empower yourself because you are no longer allowing life to run away from you. Instead, you are taking control, which has so many exciting implications. If you have the power to create pain, negativity, and hardship, you have as much power to create positivity, gratitude, and health. You have the power to create an incredible life and live it.

In my case, frequent prayer and surrender helped me through cancer. When I was diagnosed, I did not ask God to take the cancer away; the disease was mine to fix. However, I did ask for help and guidance. While I knew I had the strength to overcome this illness, I could not do it on my own. **In exchange for this guidance, I promised to be alert and aware, and to accept signs that God and the universe sent my way.**

When I started witnessing these graces, I opened myself up to the new possibilities they directed me toward. For example, I never expected to use certain treatments, like cannabis, but deciding to try everything was my ultimate test of leaving no stone unturned. By letting God guide me, I acquired a limitless way of thinking.

BELIEVE IN YOUR TREATMENT

"Respirez... Tout ira bien...BELIEVE.
Breathe...Everything will be fine...BELIEVE."

—VERONICA VILLANUEVA

You also need to believe in your treatments, not in your prognosis. Do not listen to the statistics the doctors and books tell you. Instead, focus on how your treatments will heal you. How are they affecting your body? How do they make you feel?

I knew what I needed to do to heal and I believed in my treatments, but I also felt a disconnect between that belief and the process of getting scans. From going to the hospital and getting a CT scan to then waiting for days to hear about the results, the entire process was stressful. I drove myself crazy worrying about the results from my quarterly scans. Whenever I had a test, I would rush home and obsessively check online for the message from my doctor telling me what they found.

I quickly realized I could not allow my mood and sanity to rise and fall depending on the scan results. I learned to listen to the way my body *felt* after treatments and on a daily basis. Eventually, I stopped stressing about the scan results. I made a conscious decision to not let test results rule my life and put in the effort to be more at ease. I practiced self-control by deliberately scheduling my scans on a Thursday, knowing I had to wait the whole weekend to receive my scan results the following week.

Yes, intentionally drawing out my wait seems crazy, but I have since learned to feel comfortable in uncomfortable situations. It was not easy in the beginning, but now, I often challenge and confidently tell myself "bring it on" whenever I am faced with challenges in my life. Now, challenges excite me because I know I will be a better version of myself after I learn the lesson that is put in front of me.

If you are waiting for a scan result to know whether you will live or die, you clearly have not made the decision to live. You still lack self-belief and belief in your treatments. When I began purposely scheduling my scans, I started developing my muscle of belief and muscle of surrender. I did everything I could while accepting that I could not control everything.

Now, I empower my body for each scan. If I live a full, happy, and healthy life, I know this will reflect in the scan. In fact, my belief muscle is so strong that I no longer get scans every quarter. As long as I feel as healthy as I do every day, I would rather lessen my radiation exposure than get confirmation from the scans.

Know that it may take time to build up the confidence in surrendering and belief you need to schedule your scans further apart without feeling significant stress. It took me three years to reach the point where I could avoid quarterly scans. However, over those three years, I have constantly been strengthening my belief muscle.

BELIEVE IN THE PEOPLE ADVISING YOU

"It is not so much our friends' help that helps us as it is, as the confidence of their help."

—EPICURUS

Throughout your healing journey, there should be a few people whose opinions matter to you. Think of this as your VIP list of people you trust to give you advice. Whom you include on the list is your decision; nobody deserves or is owed a spot on your list. Choose people who believe in your ability to beat your disease and who make you feel good. Remember, your mind is a powerful source of healing when you reject negative thoughts, so you need to surround yourself with positive and empowering influences, including the people around you.

For example, I rarely discussed my treatments with anyone other than my naturopathic doctors. Other people who did not understand or support my choices had no business being part of the conversation, and I did not want to spend my energy arguing with them. A key part of your transformation is to surrender control over what other people think about you and your choices. In my case, I could not control what my daughters were thinking when I decided to fight the cancer. They did not agree with some of my decisions, like to cut out sugar, but I did not let them make my decisions for me.

Everyone in your life will have an opinion about what you

should do, but you cannot listen to them all. Just like everyone has an idea of what a good mom should be, everyone has their thoughts about cancer. Instead, choose your VIP list of people whose opinions you value and believe in their ability to support you. You are not obligated to follow all their advice, but you should seek their thoughts when you need insight or a second opinion. Believe that they want the best for you.

The list of people I decided to listen to was extremely short. It consisted of my naturopathic doctors, who were giving me my treatments, and myself. **I did not require validation from anybody else.**

CHANNEL YOUR ENERGY INTO YOUR BELIEFS

"Whatever your mind can conceive and believe, it can achieve."
—NAPOLEON HILL

Believing in yourself and loving yourself go hand in hand. In fact, one of the first ways to show yourself love is to believe in yourself.

When you are first diagnosed, it can feel like you need to rush to find answers, but you have options and time. I understand that this could sound counter-intuitive, but it is true. Let me repeat this—you have options and time! Building up your muscle of belief will not happen overnight.

Transformation is a series of baby steps that has no end as long as you continue to evolve. It is a lifelong journey that will continue long after you beat cancer.

To create lasting change in your life, put energy into the things you believe in. Invest time and effort into self-improvement and your treatments. Soon enough, you will notice a ripple effect as your awareness of yourself and the world around you heightens. Everything around you will begin to align with your belief.

Have you ever noticed that when you want something, you start to see it everywhere you go? For example, imagine you desperately want a red car. Suddenly, you start recognizing red cars all around you. The reality is those red cars have always been there, but you were not yet awakened to that realization. Your awareness allows you to see the world through a different lens. Congratulations, *you* are no longer sleepwalking through life.

Once you are living in a space of self-belief and heightened awareness, you own your life. You meet the sort of people you want to meet; you see the things you want to see.

Recently, one of my clients complained that she only meets jerks when dating. Determined to help her meet different people, I encouraged her to write down a list of qualities she wants in a man. We considered how realistic those requirements were and how much she would be willing to compromise. The more she started practicing this approach, the fewer jerks she came across. Soon enough, she became so picky that her requirements were no longer realistic, and we had to shift her mindset once more.

The second you start focusing on what you believe in, the less you will see the world in your old, limiting ways. You will not see a cancer diagnosis as a death sentence; you will see it as a life sentence that lends an **opportunity to change your life.**

REDEFINING YOUR LIFE THROUGH HEALING

"The wound is the place where the Light enters you."

—RUMI

As you work through this book, you are rewriting your blueprint of what *your* healthy life should be. The more you apply this blueprint to your everyday life, the more you will master it and make it a reality.

Once you believe in yourself and your goals, you will be on the path to healing. You will notice signs from God and the universe that will reinforce your belief until it is deep in your bones.

At this point in my life, I rarely experience doubt. When I

do start to feel insecure, I think back to the last time I had confidence and succeeded. The more you live your life in this direction, the more stories you will amass to support your belief and confidence. If you ever do feel insecure, you can retrieve those stories to reignite your fate.

Doubt is normal, as is fear. These can never be eliminated, but they can be lessened. When doubt happens, you can flex your muscles of belief, hope, and strength to deal with that insecurity. As your muscles get stronger, pushing through your fear becomes easier.

With practice, your default way of thinking becomes empowered. You will no longer be living on negative and fearful autopilot. This is a game changer!

In my life, I see cancer as a detail, not a defining factor. As soon as I learned to heal my past issues—the pain, sadness, and anxiety I experienced for years during my unhappy marriage—I knew I was destined to live an incredible life. Healing had a ripple effect in that I not only beat the cancer in my body, but I improved every other aspect of my life as well. Cancer is my grace. Cancer is the road to *your* transformation.

Believing in yourself is a nonnegotiable step in the healing process because *your* mind needs to align with *your* body to make your decision to live a reality. You are the key figure in the equation, but your journey will be much easier if you have other people who support you, too.

Now that you believe in yourself and your decision to live, who will join you?

JOURNAL EXERCISE: REMEMBER
WHEN YOUR BELIEF MANIFESTED

Journaling is an important tool to reinforce your beliefs and cleanse your mind of negative thoughts. It is a practice that empowers you to feel safe to ask yourself daily questions that will lead you to live life more consciously. I journal all the time because it is a great way to release any negativity clouding my mind, especially first thing in the morning. Did you know that most of our negativity comes from recycled thoughts? They tend to be the same small group of thoughts we ruminate on over and over, filling our heads. By downloading these toxic thoughts to your journal, you can process them and not allow them to follow you throughout the day.

I understand that self-belief is easier for some people and harder for others. As a young child, I always believed in myself, but many people suffer from self-doubt. If you are struggling with self-belief, I encourage you to **pinpoint a moment in your life when you believed in yourself and received a positive outcome because of it**. Write about the experience in your journal with as much detail as you can remember. As you move forward, hold on to that memory as a reminder of your capability to make your dream outcome a reality.

Building up your confidence and belief in yourself is not an easy process. You will discover parts of yourself that you might not feel comfortable sharing with those closest to you. Think of your journal as a therapist. Your journal does not judge or talk back to you. The process can be calming, and it allows you to put things into perspective.

Your journal is an important step towards self-discovery. Through journaling, you can identify the kind of life you want to live. You can recognize your weaknesses and wake up the muscles of belief—the muscles you need to beat cancer—which have been dormant within you.

Chapter 3

SUPPORT

FIND YOUR ANGELS

"Alone, we can do so little; together, we can do so much."

—HELEN KELLER

The people around you will shape your journey in one of two ways: they will either support you and bolster your positive mindset or increase your stress and hinder your ability to heal. Therefore, the next step in your journey is to form a team of family and friends who support your decision to live and your belief in yourself.

You need two different sources of support: medical support from your doctors and emotional support from loved ones. Together, these sources will ensure your body *and* mind receive the support and care they need to work in tandem to heal you.

ASSEMBLING YOUR MEDICAL CARE TEAM

"Now faith is confidence in what we hope for and assurance about what we do not see."

—HEBREWS 11:1

When you have cancer, everybody comes to your side, which is a beautiful thing. However, you need more than well-meaning people on your support team—you need people aligned with your goals. You should not feel like you must commit to the first doctor who evaluates you. Do your research and find the best oncologist and cancer clinic for you and your goals.

This is your battle, and you get to decide the people you want to fight alongside you. This team is *yours* to assemble.

To get the best treatment possible, you want to find doctors who are on the same page as you as far as your decision to live. For example, you do not want a doctor whose top priority is end-of-life pain treatment when you are determined to beat your illness. They will not recommend the treatments you need to pursue your goal—to live.

In the early days after my diagnosis, I went through five different doctors before I found the right oncologist for me. The first five insisted I was just another statistic, which I refused to believe. They did not believe I could live. They gave me absolutely no hope.

CHEMOTHERAPY HAS ITS PLACE

I want to be clear that I am not against chemotherapy. In fact, I think it is the right option in certain cases. However, I do believe chemotherapy should be partnered with something to balance, equip, and empower your body and immune system.

If your doctor recommends chemotherapy or radiation, *do not reject it out of hand!* Any concerns you have about chemical treatments need to be a conversation you have with your doctor. Your doctor can address how chemotherapy will impact your particular illness and situation.

Now that I have more knowledge, I understand why I did not qualify for chemotherapy. In my case, the cancer had metastasized, which meant it had spread and could not be targeted with chemotherapy. The tumors plagued my upper body, and chemotherapy would not have been able to eliminate them. Your situation may be different from mine.

After I went to the emergency room, numerous doctors visited me and compared opinions about my situation. They could not make sense of my blood results, which were somewhat normal despite the clear presence of cancer in my scans. They drained 1.6 liters of fluid from my right lung. Before they performed a biopsy, they had already diagnosed me. In fact, the doctor told my daughters before I had even woken up from my surgery that I did not qualify for chemotherapy or radiotherapy.

At the time, I did not fully understand what the doctors

meant. *Why on Earth would they not treat the cancer?* Later, I realized what they were really saying: "It is too late for these treatments to help." Tumors had plagued my upper body so telling them to cure me was undoubtedly an impossible and unreasonable demand!

I decided to view their decision to forego chemotherapy and radiation as grace. It was a blessing; God gave me this cancer and my only option for fighting it was through natural means. In a way, that decision spared me from needing to further stress my body with more toxins. The fact that I had to deeply believe in life and my ability to beat cancer were gifts because it made me develop the positive mindset I have carried with me even after recovering—a mindset that has made me a believer and a more compassionate, optimistic person. Had circumstances been different, my doctors might have pressured me to do chemotherapy instead of understanding that healing my mental and emotional wounds was connected to healing my physical body.

FINDING THE RIGHT DOCTOR FOR ME

"We must not allow other people's limited perceptions to define us."

—VIRGINIA SATIR

It took rejecting five doctors until I finally found one who *did* believe in me. Naturally, he became an important member of my support team.

When I first met my oncologist at UCLA, he never told me I had six months to live, unlike previous doctors. He explained that I was at stage 4, which meant the cancer had metastasized. I liked how he wanted to educate me without passing any judgment. Although he made the facts clear, he did not give me a death sentence. This doctor offered options, which gave me hope.

Over the years, the trust and understanding between my oncologist and me have grown. He never tells me what to do; he performs my scans and interprets the results. He respects and commends me for my strength without getting too involved in the details of the treatments I undergo with my naturopathic doctors. When I meet with him, he interprets my scan, asks me how I am doing, and encourages me to continue doing whatever it is I am doing. In fact, he gives me the green light to do all the things I want to do, and most importantly, the things I need to *be happy*! Above that, he asks *me* when *I* want to have a scan. He spends no time convincing me of what I should be doing, just like I waste no time convincing him of my methods, many of which fall outside the realm of conventional Western medicine. This is what it means to BELIEVE in ME!

In fact, the only time he ever offered me advice was in front of my daughter, when he told me that I did not have to stop eating sugar or animal protein. At the time, I had lost so much weight that I was down to eighty-nine pounds. I did not waste energy arguing with him because I understood his comments came from a place of concern, but I was fighting my own battle, so I put my energy into that.

As you search for doctors, be selective about who you choose to support and treat you. As I have mentioned before, all your energy should go towards your own healing. Anything that drains your energy, like conflict and pushback from other people, including your doctor, should be eliminated from your life.

IDENTIFYING YOUR EMOTIONAL CHEERLEADERS

"Friends are the siblings God never gave us."

—MENCIUS

When I first learned about my diagnosis, I never expected my friends to become the powerful supportive force they turned out to be. Throughout my journey, they have been my biggest emotional supporters—my cheerleaders and angels.

As empowered people themselves, my friends understood my decision to live and my belief in myself, and they have never treated me like a victim. In fact, they encouraged me to continue being a warrior and keep fighting hard. I chose friends who aligned with my beliefs. I deeply believe that the friends I have are yet another way God is saying, "You are not alone in this journey."

As my life changed, so did my circle of friends. Cancer is a real change, and it exposed who my true friends are. Surround yourself with the people in your life who believe in you. You may be surprised who steps up and who lets you down. If someone acts as a negative influence on you by discouraging you or criticizing your decisions, you may need to distance yourself from them. You can still listen to what they have to say, but you do not need to follow their advice. Although they might care about you, chances are they are coming from a place of fear. Their recommendations or beliefs are made out of their own fears—for example, a fear that you will struggle and suffer, like the fear my daughters had for me—which gets projected onto you. You cannot spend time trying to change those people because when you are fighting for your life, you do not have that kind of energy to spare.

If someone is not on your list of supporters, you do not need to alienate yourself from them completely. They are still part of your world. Instead, you must exercise your muscles of resilience, strength, and belief in yourself. Different people will induce different emotions within you, including fear, helplessness, and disbelief, even if they mean well. Your responsibility is either to muscle up or create the necessary boundary for your own success.

FAMILY DOES NOT GUARANTEE SUPPORT

"It's your life. Don't let anyone make you feel guilty for living it your way."

—UNKNOWN

To succeed in your healing journey, you need to detox your mind of any negative thoughts. Often, this also means detoxing your external environment by removing any pessimistic people who drain your energy. As I said, you do not need to cut people out of your life forever, but you may need some temporary distance. They should not take this personally. As I said, you need to do what is right for *you*!

My friends turned out to be more supportive than I expected, but the opposite happened with my family. After my diagnosis, I did not see my mother for several months because I knew she had a more negative outlook on my prognosis than I did. If I had allowed her to be around me, she would have spent her time crying, and I did not want to be surrounded by sadness and negativity. At the time, I needed to be my own advocate. I chose to be open and honest with my mother. My decision to distance myself was not about her, it was about me. I needed to do what was right for me, which meant surrounding myself with empowering and uplifting people. As hard as this was for my mother, she understood that this was not a personal attack on her, and that the priority was for her daughter to get well. She respected my decision and supported me by praying for me. This was enough for me.

Distancing myself from my mother taught me how important it is to set healthy boundaries. Creating boundaries was something new for me, especially towards my mother and children. Having boundaries during an illness is self-love. They are necessary, and everyone around you needs to respect them. So, why is it hard for us to set healthy boundaries, especially towards people we love? The fear of losing their love and the fear of them being angry at us sometimes holds us back from setting the boundaries we need. The advice I have for you is to prioritize yourself over everyone else. It sounds harsh and mean, but you should not be around people who expect you to prioritize *them* but are unwilling to prioritize *you*.

A natural part of your healing process is to have a clean life, which requires eliminating toxic people who bring you down. To be clear, my mother is not a bad person. I know she loves me and wants all of this to go away. Negative people are not necessarily acting maliciously. They simply cannot control the negative energy they put out, which for the most part, they are not even aware of emitting.

If someone cannot support you in your healing stage while

you are trying to establish an empowering environment, you should not have them in your life until you can set those healthy boundaries.

I did not ban my mother from coming to see me. Instead, I set a boundary to stop myself from suffering. I explained to her that **I could not fight her**, so she had to respect everything I was doing, even if it did not make sense to her.

We grow up conditioned to believe that our families always know and want the best thing for us. I no longer believe that. **Your family loves you, but you are the *only* person who knows what is best for you.**

Throughout this process, you should never have to justify your actions. My oncologist never asked me to justify the treatments I chose to do, which is why I included him on my support team. Justifications are a waste of energy. Remember, people can be supportive of you without fully understanding what you are doing. You cannot expect everyone to understand. Equally, you cannot expect validation for all your choices.

ISOLATION IS DANGEROUS

"Walking with a friend in the dark is better than walking alone in the light."

—HELEN KELLER

You might wonder, *if people will criticize and judge my choices, do I need to be around them at all?*

You need other people because, as I discussed earlier, you must continue living a fulfilling life throughout your treatment. If you shut yourself off from the world, you will wither away. Science backs up the assertion that social support facilitates healing. **When people feed you love, the hormone associated with happiness, oxytocin, is released in your body.** Not only does this hormone naturally reduce stress but it is an anti-depressant and is anti-anxiety. To maximize your body's ability to heal, surround yourself with angels who can give you love, inspire hope, and build your strength.

One of my favorite and most sacred moments is when I encounter like-minded people and have profound, mind-blowing conversations. Do you know when you are with or talking with the right people? When you leave them, you feel amazing and exhilarated. You feel understood. This type of connection is key to my happiness.

Ever since my diagnosis, I decided to design my new life like a tourist in the City of Angels. I love living in Los Angeles! I have the canyons half a mile from me, Santa Monica beach thirty minutes away, and a short two-and-a-half-hour drive to the magical mountains and desert. I am blessed that no matter where I go, I easily meet incredible people who have added joy and happiness to my life.

Whatever you do, avoid isolation. The more you surround yourself with family, friends, and allies who promote healing, the better you will feel emotionally and physically. Being fed love is an important part of your healing process, as is the love you feed yourself.

When people receive a difficult diagnosis, they tend to isolate themselves. This is not a healthy approach. Not only do you need to continue, but you need to start living the life that you envisioned when you decided to live. Every day you are paving the path towards that life.

OPEN YOURSELF AND ACCEPT SUPPORT

"The reason I'm being positive is to make everyone around me to get the positive energy."

—SIVAPRAKASH SIDHU

For many years, I generously gave my support to other people. After my diagnosis, it was my turn to receive help. One of my best friends encouraged me to accept that support willingly, instead of feeling like a burden to those around me. "We know you're strong," she said. "You're probably such a badass, you can do this on your own. But it's time for you to surrender and let us help you. Let us be your rock, as well."

Asking for support does *not* make you weak. Quite the

opposite, in fact. To ask for help and support requires strength and courage. It is an important lesson in humility. Open yourself up to any help that comes your way.

It will be very hard to get support if you refuse to talk about what you are going through. This is your first lesson in vulnerability. Do not be ashamed by the cancer in your body. The worst thing you can do is not talk about the disease in your body. Instead of suppressing it, acknowledge it. Talk to people. **How do you expect anyone to support you if they do not know what you need from them?**

The way I see it, we are never going to make progress in the subject of cancer if we keep our stories to ourselves. In writing this book, my hope is that opening up about the disease in my body will help others to share their own story. We need to learn from each other's experiences. Cancer should not be your secret; see it as your grace in your life.

There are multiple ways to give and receive support, and they all begin with talking to others about your experience. For example, I found my naturopathic doctor from a stranger whose best friend survived cancer because of her. **I found my Western oncologist by asking people *I* knew to talk to people *they* knew about recommendations.**

The more you share information about yourself, the more you widen the pool of people working to help you. By speaking out, you widen your support system, often in the most unexpected ways.

SUPPORT FROM FRIENDS

The following excerpt is from one of my conversations with my best friend, Lauren, in her words:

Early on, right after you were diagnosed at Eisenhower and were recovering in your Palm Desert home, you said you weren't ready for your mom to visit you. When I asked why, you said that she would see you as a victim. She would ask, "Why you? Why would this happen to *you*?"

You looked at me and said, "Why not me? Why shouldn't I get this?"

While you may have been unable to fully articulate your thoughts on this, you were already developing the concept that there's a reason you were given cancer.

In another conversation, you told me you believed you were given cancer to make you stronger, to learn life lessons, etc. I told you that I would have a chat with God and let him know that you no longer needed any character-building exercises—that, really, you were good! Your character was sufficiently built!

In the early days following the discovery of the cancer, when doctors told you that the cancer was so advanced you had only six months to live, you told them, "That just means we have a lot of wood to chop?"

You said, "If cancer thought it was going to defeat me, it chose the wrong body!"

MAGIC HAPPENS IN UNEXPECTED PLACES

"Your acts of kindness are iridescent wings of divine love, which linger and continue to uplift others long after your sharing."

—RUMI

When you surrender to the Universe and God, an amazing thing happens: you find support and answers in the most unexpected places.

I had created a dating profile on the website Match.com, but after my diagnosis, dating was the last thing on my mind. Still, my profile showed up as active on the website. I only thought about it because a notification popped up on my phone every time a guy liked my profile. I told myself, "I should turn this off," but something told me not to.

Now, I know the reason why. The universe and God had something in store for me—**a sign** that led me toward my naturopathic doctor who played a major role in my healing process.

A few weeks after receiving my diagnosis, instead of deleting my profile and trying to hide the cancer diagnosis, I put it all out there. **As I have said, it's important not to feel ashamed of cancer and think of yourself as a victim, because if you hide it, the disease will stay inside you.** Instead, reverse and replace that mindset. Think about all the people who would support you if you told them what you were going through.

I edited my profile and wrote, *I have to get off this app for a bit because I was just diagnosed with cancer. No worries. I'll be back with an even better version of me!*

I found humor in the situation and ended my profile message with *message me only if you have a joke that would make me laugh.*

What followed was an incredible outpouring of men sending me encouraging messages, emojis of flowers, and notes that said, "I'm praying for you." I felt the compassion of people despite not knowing them. This reinforced my belief in the innate compassion and goodness of people. Remember this: you do not need to know the people praying for you.

The power of prayers, *even* from strangers, is a gift. I had so many people praying for me, and truthfully speaking, I felt it. Talk about support! When you're healing, you need as much support as you can get, not only from the people closest to you but from people you don't even know. There is power in people praying for you, no matter who or where they are. I was graced by so many people praying for me.

Among the notes of support, one man messaged me to say a friend of his had recovered from cancer after seeing a naturopathic doctor. Some people would have called me crazy for listening to a stranger, but part of opening yourself up to all possibilities is being non-judgmental and believing in people. I thought, *why would this stranger want to harm me?* I believed he genuinely wanted to help. As humans, we can't just turn our backs on human suffering.

I contacted the doctor he recommended, and ever since, she has been my doctor. I found the help I needed thanks to that man and my willingness to listen to strangers—at the time they were strangers, now I believe they are my angels sent by the higher power.

As Anaïs Nin said, "Life shrinks or expands in proportion to one's courage."

To live through your illness and come out a better version of yourself, you need to remain open to every possibility. Look for the signs in your life. I interpreted that man's message as a sign, and it led me to the doctor I needed to treat me.

A good doctor-patient match goes both ways. I connected with mine instantly, and I believe the feeling was mutual, as she describes in her own words in the following excerpt.

DOCTOR'S VOICE: MEETING VERONICA

"I am blessed to be a part of Veronica's (or V, as I call her) cancer journey—and it has been quite a ride. To best appreciate how incredible this woman is, I will be highlighting her medical care and treatment protocols that brought her to where she is today.

"I first met V through the most unusual referral source of my career, Match.com. No, we didn't match each other's profiles. However, a past patient of mine saw V's health update on her profile and threw my name out there and it stuck. I saw V for the first time two months after her diagnosis, on November 23, 2016. V came in with her best friend, Emily, to help with remembering her visit and treatment instructions.

"V was extremely weak, fatigued, in pain, and cachectic (her body was wasting away), but her spirit was alive and kicking. Her diagnosis was stage 4 lung cancer and her prognosis was less than a year. What I remember most of our first meeting was the fire in her eyes and the absolute certainty that she would not be defeated and would come through her diagnosis. The first thing she told me was that she would only work with doctors who believed that she would live. She wanted to do everything she could to make it happen, and I was determined to walk this path with her."

SIGNS OF GRACE: MY HUMMINGBIRD MESSENGER

"There are only two ways to live your life: as though nothing is a miracle, or as though everything is a miracle."

—MAHATMA GANDHI

The positive people in your life will give you much-needed support, but so will the universe, if you let it. Once you start believing in yourself and a higher power, you begin seeing signs of the universe's support everywhere you go.

The last time I visited San Francisco, I was in a building in the city with the window cracked open four inches. I spoke with a religious friend of mine, Kathy, whom I had not seen since my diagnosis, and she asked me if I had prayed. I told her that, even though I, myself, and everyone I knew were praying for me, I had not explicitly asked God to take the cancer away. I only asked for signs to guide me in the right direction.

The second I said the word "sign," a hummingbird flew in through the four-inch opening of the window, on the ninth floor, and gently touched my cheek. Moments later, the bird flew back out again.

Afterward, Kathy hugged me and said, "There is your sign."

She told me that God had sent the hummingbird to reassure me that I was going to be just fine. This was such a sacred moment for me. I don't think Kathy knew what she had given me by interpreting what we just witnessed. She gave me hope, and as I have said before, *hope* is the best gift one can give to someone who has been diagnosed with a terminal disease.

I believe in these words said by Napoleon Bonaparte: "There is no such thing as accident; it is fate misnamed."

Ever since that moment, a hummingbird has been my sign.

When I shared this beautiful moment with my best friend, Emily, who is a spiritual person, she looked up the meaning behind hummingbirds. We learned angels send them as messengers of joy and all things good. The bird symbolizes courage, determination, and adaptability. Although extremely light in weight, a hummingbird has the courage of a lion!

This was the first of many times a hummingbird would visit me. I received another visit from this bird the first night after I moved to a new place in Los Angeles. I had opened all the windows and sliding doors in the house because I love the feeling of being surrounded by nature and breathing fresh air.

You can guess what happened next. My angel sent another hummingbird with another message.

Pete, whom I consider my brother, and who accompanies me to all my scans, was with me at the time. As I showed him around my place, a hummingbird flew in and welcomed me in my new home. No matter how hard we tried, the bird did not want to leave.

Two years later, I had to move from that home. I found a new house in the hills, which I loved. The home had a peaceful, quiet, and positive energy. This is where I gave birth to *The Grace of Cancer*.

Despite loving the new house, I had not committed to moving yet. As I debated whether to make the move, a hummingbird visited me again. It sat on a sculpture hanging directly above my head. Later that evening, as I prepared to go to dinner with my friends, the hummingbird was still there. I told the bird it had to leave so I could close the doors, but no matter what I did, it would not go. I had to leave, but I did not want the bird to feel trapped.

"If somebody burglarizes me, so be it. You're in charge now," I said to the bird. I left all the sliding doors open so it could breathe.

When I returned home around eleven o'clock at night, the bird was waiting for me, right by the front door. As I walked up the stairs, the bird followed me all the way to my bedroom. Nobody had robbed my house while I was out with friends. Thank God!

When I woke up the next morning, the hummingbird was gone. Pete, interpreting the visit, told me the bird first came to reassure me that I had made the right choice to live there two years ago. Not only did the bird stay with me overnight to make sure I was okay, but to give me clarity on my decision to move to the hills and leave West Holly-wood. I believed the hummingbird was encouraging me to make this change that I was reluctant to make. It would be a better home and environment for me to write my book. The bird was absolutely right as I love living near Runyon Canyon, making it my special place where I have done most of my creative thinking and introspective reflections.

Because of these signs, I am convinced that my first support system is God and the universe. I live my life according to the spiritual guidance I am given. Now, when I have a dilemma, I ask the universe for answers. Most of the time, the answers we need are right there in front of us, but we are usually too busy and distracted to notice them. You need to slow down and open yourself up to receiving guidance. This requires being in the moment.

As James Russell Lowell said, "Fate loves the fearless."

My sign, the hummingbird, and the positive people in my

life helped me feel the support I needed to let go of my fear, uncertainty, and anxiety. No human is fearless, and I am not ashamed to admit that after my diagnosis, fear occupied my mind. Throughout your journey, you will find your own signs, which will turn your fear into excitement, as well as other coping mechanisms, like channeling your energy into education.

JOURNAL EXERCISE: CREATE YOUR LIST OF SUPPORTERS

For this chapter's journal exercise, I would like you to make a list of all the people you interact with on a regular basis. Now, remove any people from your list who are negative influences. Who criticizes or discourages you? Who depletes your energy? Who does not believe in you and your decisions?

Narrow your list down further. Who makes you feel supported? Happy? Loved?

These people are your angels and cheerleaders. When you feel alone or isolated, revisit this list. Reach out to the people you trust to support you and draw strength from their love.

Chapter 4

EDUCATION

EMPOWER YOURSELF WITH KNOWLEDGE

"Knowledge is power."

—SIR FRANCIS BACON

Once you start the journey of learning about cancer and understanding the type affecting you, the knowledge you gain takes your mind off the emotional part of having this disease. You won't feel afraid, anxious, or like a victim anymore. You will have no room in your head for those negative emotions. Instead, you will feel empowered.

Information is power, especially when followed by **massive** actions. When you are first diagnosed, you don't know where to start, but by studying the disease, you learn you have options. You fill your brain with information on how to promote healing. Trust me, once you know the steps you can take to protect and nourish your body, you will be excited to apply them. Hopefully, you feel the same excitement and empowerment from reading this book and hearing my story.

When I received my diagnosis, reading, studying, and listening to audiobooks made me feel empowered. I decided to be proactive and educate myself, and the more I learned, the more I knew I could reverse the cancer. I already believed I was going to live and be healthier than ever, but now I had science-backed reasons reinforcing my belief. I discovered the treatments I needed to pursue: detoxing, eating green vegetables, getting enough sleep, and more, which you'll learn about in the following chapters. By understanding the disease and my health, I felt in control and confident that I could reverse the disease.

TAKING ACTION WITH EDUCATION

"Don't let your learning lead to knowledge. Let your learning lead to action."

—JIM ROHN

Deciding to live is not enough without belief, support, and action. When you choose to live, you have to actually **do** something about it. You have work to do! When I chose to live, I simultaneously chose to educate myself. I would wake up every day and sit at my computer ordering books, reading, and calling doctors. By spending each day in research mode, I had no time to view myself as a victim.

Alternatively, if someone has been diagnosed with cancer and they decide to live, but they stay at home all day wallowing and obsessing over their diagnosis, they will not make progress. While that person might have decided to live, they are not moving forward in any productive way. Their actions are not aligned with their decision.

The decision alone is not enough. **To make your decisions come to life, you need actions.**

FEED YOUR MIND: DATA GATHERING

"Education breeds confidence. Confidence breeds hope. Hope breeds peace."

—CONFUCIUS

In the same way we feed our stomachs with the right food, we can feed our brains with information that promotes a positive and healing mindset. The type of research you do will shape your outlook. Make sure to read books that *empower* you. If you read a well-credited book that encourages you to live and asserts that healing is possible, you will have a much more positive view on your situation than if you only read depressing statistics. I have included a **recommended reading list in Appendix A.**

Educating yourself on your disease allows you to better understand your options for treatment while also keeping your mind from wandering.

A wandering mind is dangerous because by not releasing negative thoughts, you can quickly spiral into depression or anxiety. Remember, humans are programmed to ruminate on worst-case scenarios. When you focus on the past, you become depressed. Our default is to worry. When you worry about the future, it creates anxiety. If we are not worrying about today, we are likely worrying about tomorrow. The key is to stay present and focused. Be in the moment, and you will be graced with such an alertness and clarity that will allow you to see the gifts of being in the present.

The more you focus on education, the less your mind will wander into the world of toxicity. Educating yourself is a foolproof way for your mind to stay focused on positive action.

BABY STEPS IN THE RIGHT DIRECTION

"The journey of a thousand miles begins with one step."

—LAO TZU

Your journey will take you to the top of a mountain, so baby steps are better than standing still. Create excitement for yourself by researching all the treatments available for your particular type of cancer. When I learned more about the disease in my body, I could not wait to meet another doctor to discuss treatments or try incorporating a different food into my diet. Learning about my options made me feel like I was doing something productive, instead of merely sitting around and doing nothing.

Throughout this process, I encourage you to leave your comfort zone behind. Be open to other treatments that are not necessarily the conventional methods being recommended by Western oncologists.

The more open-minded you are in your research, the more options will become available to you.

ASKING THE RIGHT QUESTIONS

When you receive a prognosis, it is important to ask the right questions:

- What type of cancer is it?
- Where is the original source of the disease in my body?
- Where is the tumor(s) located in my body?
- What stage has the cancer reached?
- Has it metastasized?

With the answers to these questions, you can understand the characteristics of the cancer and how likely it is to grow or spread. For example, the type of cancer I had would likely have traveled to my brain next.

My research led me from one question to the next. After researching the science behind cancer, I thought of my internal terrain like a fish tank filled with murky water. From there, I started researching how to balance my body. I learned that my body must be pH balanced. pH stands for power hydrogen, which is a measurement of hydrogen ions in our bodies. The ideal pH lies between 7.30 and 7.45. Anything below this range means the body is in an acidic state.

When I gained this knowledge, I immediately wanted to test the acidity in my body. I had nothing to lose by gaining more knowledge and data. I obtained a package of litmus paper and tested my urine first thing in the morning, before eating or drinking anything.

Instantly, I had a shocking result: The acidity levels in my body measured off the chart. Knowing the harmful effects of an overly acidic body, I became obsessed with making my body alkalinized—the opposite of acidic. Testing my internal pH level became part of my regular routine.

The great French scientist Antoine Béchamp once said, "The germ is nothing; the terrain is everything."

In other words, harmful bacteria and pathogens in the body do not determine your overall health, whereas the balance of cellular pH in the body has a significant impact on your disease state. Judging by that quote, Antoine Béchamp has a more holistic approach to medicine, as he believed that the internal environment makes one sick, rather than the external circumstances. As long as your body's internal ecosystem remains healthy and balanced, your immune system can handle any germ that comes your way.

Personally, I found this idea more compelling than the theories of Louis Pasteur, who famously advocated that disease comes from one's external environment.

While I agree with Pasteur insofar as my unhappy external environment affected my health, I believe the way I internally processed that environment is what made me sick. My research led me to conclude that I developed cancer because my internal systems fell out of balance.

If your immune system is weakened, you will get sick. As Béchamp says, it is all about your internal terrain. Before I could start to heal, I needed to do everything I could to balance my pH level and eliminate the toxins in my body, which essentially led me to detoxification.

Remember, the mind influences the body and, therefore, helps shape your internal terrain.

THE HOLISTIC APPROACH

"If you are going through hell, keep going."

—WINSTON CHURCHILL

When my research led me to an alternative way of thinking about illness, I decided to pursue that path of treatment. Why? The idea that *I* could reverse the disease empowered me. The holistic approach, which involves treating underlying issues in the body and mind through non-pharmacological methods, offered more hope than the conventional path. After all, conventional Western doctors told me I had six months to live. Alternative treatments, which I'll explore in greater depth in the coming chapters, were my only path forward. I became obsessed with finding approaches that would allow my body to heal naturally.

Focus your research on results. Thanks to the internet, it is easier to do research today than ever before. The downside to easily available information is that there are many conflicting ideas out there. For this reason, I advise you to be careful not to become overwhelmed by information. The idea is not to uncover the root cause of cancer. If you already have cancer, focus on the question "what can I do to get rid of the cancer?" not "why did I get it?" In this process of studying and getting rid of the disease, you will uncover the cause of your cancer.

In my case, the cancer had metastasized. I wanted to reduce

the number of tumors I had, so I researched how to achieve that result and focused all my energy on making it happen. *My goal was never to research the cause of cancer; my mission was always to heal myself.*

If you feel stuck and don't know what your next steps should be, research can point you in the right direction. Educating yourself makes you fluid, flowing, and moving forward toward a solution instead of stuck in inaction. Reading this book is a great first step!

BELIEF IS THE NEW SUPERPOWER

"I believe in intuitions and inspirations...I sometimes FEEL that I am right. I do not KNOW that I am."

—ALBERT EINSTEIN

Remember, **choosing to live means choosing to take action.** I set a goal for myself to make every day exciting. Even at my sickest period, I still woke up, put on makeup, and styled my hair because those steps were an important part of self-care for me. Your self-care routine might look different from mine—what is important is to stick with yours. When you choose to live, choose *not* to live an unconscious and mediocre life! Be alive! Do more than exist on autopilot.

Many people die from cancer before they have actually

died from the disease. They die a metaphorical, emotional, and spiritual death. The best medicine for that disease is education and lifestyle. The more you learn about the tremendous progress in the subject of cancer, the more optimistic you start to feel, and the more motivation you will have to live.

When I was first diagnosed, I had to believe that I was going to pull through. For me, that initial belief came from God, the universe, and the support system around me. Once I believed I was going to live, I started reading to reinforce that hope. By doing my research, I was not just feeling some unexplained belief, I had cold, hard facts.

Armed with knowledge, I didn't only *believe* I would get better; I *felt* it. The more you educate yourself, the more you reinforce your beliefs.

FIND BALANCE BETWEEN LOGIC AND EMOTIONS

"Asking 'why?' can lead to understanding. Asking 'why not?' can lead to breakthroughs."

—DANIEL H. PINK

Your left brain is the more logical, fact-based side of your mind, while your right brain is more emotional and intuitive. For those of you who rely on your left brain, a gut instinct will not be convincing enough to quell your doubt and anxiety, so you need education to back up your beliefs. Personally, I rely more on my right brain. For me, a feeling is enough.

Throughout history, we have been taught to pay more attention to our left brains than our right. In my opinion, we have done ourselves a disservice by not developing the emotional, intuitive muscles in our right brains. Although we have raised great mathematicians and engineers, a lot of these jobs are becoming obsolete because they can be computerized. However, you cannot write a program on how to feel.

I am not advocating to disregard our left brains entirely. As with many things, I believe in a healthy collaboration between left and right brain. Give credit to both. A state of homeostasis can exist in your body and in your mind.

A NEW, EMPOWERED YOU

"The comeback is always stronger than the setback."

—DR. JILL MURRAY

Education has the power to take "victim" out of your vocabulary. Replacing your "why" with "how" is more empowering. As you learn information, you shed the idea of being a victim. Studying, talking, and meeting other people makes you an empowered person because you learn how to take action and help yourself. Only then can you *feel* cancer as a grace and a catalyst to change your life. Only by educating yourself can you earn that experience and see grace in all the steps towards healing.

The treatment plan offered by your Western doctor is likely *not* the only treatment appropriate for your cancer. Like me, you may find the answers to your disease in alternative medicine, as we'll explore further in the next chapter.

JOURNAL EXERCISE: BECOME A NOTE TAKER

As you research your illness, take detailed notes in your journal. What treatment options do you want to pursue? Which resources have been most insightful? What facts or figures have stood out to you?

Learn to be a fastidious note taker so you can return to the valuable information you have found in the future. This habit will be especially useful when you want to ask questions or present information to your doctor.

Chapter 5

WESTERN MEDICINE AND ALTERNATIVE MEDICINE

BEST OF BOTH WORLDS

"The secret of change is to focus all of your energy not on fighting the old, but on building the new."

—DAN MILLMAN

Although my diagnosis had the word "incurable" attached to it, I never wavered from the idea that I would, one day, be healed. The reason I am here today is because I explored more than one avenue. I was committed to being open to any natural cancer therapy, regardless of how bizarre or strange it may have seemed. Not only did I regularly see a Western oncologist, but I was also treated by an integrative doctor. When I formed my medical team, I wanted to have the best of both worlds. That way, I would achieve the unthinkable—TO LIVE!

I am a firm believer that the best things in life are the result of a collaborative effort. Throughout my healing process, I chose to have **both** a Western oncologist and an integrative doctor. To get the best outcome, I took the best of both worlds. My oncologist interpreted my scans while my integrative doctor guided me through my day-to-day treatments.

One of the frustrations I have is the disconnect and unfamiliarity of Western doctors with nutritional and holistic therapies to prevent and treat cancer. A great deal of misunderstanding still exists around alternative treatments in the public sphere in that people believe the approaches are pseudoscientific "woo-woo" and not evidence-informed. We have been programmed to believe that conventional doctors know best, but the Western and integrative approaches to healing complement each other and can help you beat cancer.

I know no one better equipped to clear up the misconceptions than my own talented naturopathic doctor, who has written the following excerpt.

DOCTOR'S VOICE: UNDERSTANDING INTEGRATIVE MEDICINE

"My practice focus is on integrative oncology and regenerative medicine for joint pain and injury. What is a naturopathic doctor (ND)?

"For those of you who are not familiar with my field of medicine, let me give you a brief introduction. Naturopathic medicine originated in Europe in the 16th and 17th centuries as a traditional healing modality. It was brought to North America in the late 1800s, pioneered by Dr. Benedict Lust, from Germany. After getting my bachelor's degree from UCLA, I went to National University of Natural Medicine in Portland, Oregon (formerly National College of Naturopathic Medicine), the oldest naturopathic medical school in North America. It is a four-year postgraduate, doctoral program.

"The philosophy of naturopathic medicine is based on our body's amazing ability to heal itself with gentle support from our food, water, and medicines as needed. Instead of focusing on only symptom management, we spend time to find the root cause of the illness and treat that imbalance. In my practice, that means that I spend a lot of time with my patients, not only on their cancer treatment, but also on their everyday health practices such as what they eat, how they exercise their body, and how they detox with a healthy gut and immune function.

"I utilize an integrative approach to health and healing. In 2017, the National Cancer Institute defined 'integrative oncology' as 'a patient-centered, evidence-informed field of cancer care that utilizes mind and body practices, natural products, and/or lifestyle modifications from different traditions alongside conventional cancer treatments. Integrative oncology aims to optimize health, quality of life, and clinical outcomes across the cancer care continuum and to empower people to prevent cancer and become active participants before, during, and beyond cancer treatment.'

"The majority of my evidence-informed treatment protocols are geared towards supporting the body's innate healing response and enhancing the response toward conventional treatments. There is a time and place for all medicine. I find that my patients, like Veronica, who utilize both appropriate conventional and naturopathic care, have better tolerance and greater success with their treatment protocols."

DIFFERING PHILOSOPHIES

"We must not allow other people's limited perceptions to define us."

—VIRGINIA SATIR

A huge disconnect exists between Western treatments and holistic therapies when it comes to preventing and treating cancer.

Conventional medicine is tied up in the old belief system, which argues that illnesses arise from our genetics and biochemistry. According to Western philosophies, genetic predispositions cause cancer more than lifestyles. Statistically, fewer than 20 percent of cancer cases result from DNA damage. The other 80 percent or more are caused by poor diet and generally unhealthy lifestyles. This connection to lifestyle is known as metabolic.

According to Dr. Nasha Winters and Jess Higgins Kelley, "Study after study shows that only 5–10 percent of cancer is caused by damaged DNA[…]The remaining 90–95 percent of cancer cases are caused by poor diet and unhealthy lifestyles that also damage mitochondrial function."[2]

Integrative medicine believes that the cause of cancer is metabolic. When you believe in metabolic causes, your goal becomes to reinstate the balance of your body in order to heal. In contrast, Western medicine only looks at cancer from a genetic perspective. Many Western doctors do not believe cancer can be reversed. That is why doctors work with pharmaceutical companies to provide chemical medications to treat the disease. **This is something to take into consideration when you are evaluating your options.**

---

2   Winters, Nasha, and Jess Higgins Kelley. *The Metabolic Approach to Cancer: Integrating Deep Nutrition, the Ketogenic Diet, and Nontoxic Bio-Individualized Therapies.* White River Junction, VT: Chelsea Green Publishing, 2017.

Obviously and tragically, people do die of cancer. Despite this, it is still realistic to believe that cancer can be reversed. You can heal yourself. After all, I did.

NECESSARY LIFESTYLE CHANGES

"Progress is impossible without change, and those who cannot change their minds cannot change anything."

—GEORGE BERNARD SHAW

Cancer expert Dr. Patrick Quillin supports the argument that lifestyle accounts for most cancer cases, saying, "Lifestyle is at least 90 percent responsible for cancer, while genes play a 5–10 percent role."[3]

In my case, the cancer was not genetic. That was one of the first questions I asked after my diagnosis because I wanted to make sure my children did not have the disease, too. As soon as I knew the cancer was not genetic, I became interested in the impact of my lifestyle on my overall health.

Think of lifestyle as the crossroads of your mind, body, soul, and spirit. How you feel mentally and physically influences how you live, and vice versa.

Integrative medicine helped me look at my body holisti-

---

3   Quillin, Patrick, and Noreen Quillin. *Beating Cancer with Nutrition.* Tulsa, OK: Nutrition Times Press, 2005.

cally, as an entire system, and made me realize I had to change my lifestyle. It takes courage, discipline, consistency, and commitment to see the benefits of a holistic path to healing, but it can work for you.

Our bodies want to be healthy. While the body can genetically generate disease on its own, the biggest problem is *us* and the abuse we inflict on our bodies. In my case, I put my body under so much stress as a consequence of my unhappy marriage and subsequent divorce. My integrative doctor suggested a cortisol (stress hormone) manager to help deal with my stress levels. At the time, I also ate a ridiculous amount of sugar, which I have eliminated from my diet.

Alternative medicine promotes an integrative approach focused on lifestyle changes. Western medicine promotes pills, the side effects of which could be detrimental. The beauty of alternative treatments is that they have few to no side effects.

COMBATING CHEMOTHERAPY

"The wish for healing has always been half of health."

—LUCIUS ANNAEUS SENECA

Some people have no choice but to go through chemotherapy, which causes many negative effects like nausea and hair loss. However, by combining a Western approach (chemotherapy) with alternative therapies, you can counteract some of the symptoms and damage. For example, if you are going through chemotherapy, an integrative doctor might suggest a way to boost your immune system to minimize poisoning your body and reduce the serious side effects of radiation.

In their book *The Metabolic Approach to Cancer*, Dr. Nasha Winters and Jess Higgins Kelley explain the conventional approach to cancer:

> Leading cancer treatments such as chemotherapy and radiation are, in fact, carcinogenic, meaning they actually *cause* cancer. Indeed, several cancer drugs including tamoxifen, used to treat breast cancer, are classified by the International Agency for Research on Cancer (IARC) as Group 1 carcinogens—meaning carcinogenic in humans. So is radiation. Yet when you or the person next to you is diagnosed with cancer, then surgery, radiation, or chemotherapy, or a combination of these, will be your primary treatment options.
>
> These modalities will, in words used by those in the oncology field, "slash, burn, and poison" cancer cells in hopes of killing them. (Early chemotherapies were actually derived from mustard gas, a chemical agent of war.) The trouble is that these conventional treatments also slash, burn, and poison a body's healthy cells. Not only that, but they further deplete the

immune system, damage DNA, eradicate critical microbes in the gut, cause inflammation and oxidative stress—all of which are cancer-*promoting* factors.[4]

If you are going through chemotherapy and radiation, it is in your best interest to arm yourself with a naturopathic doctor who can help with the detoxification of your body as well as rebuilding your immune system.

When your immune system is depleted, you become more vulnerable to other illnesses. That is why chemotherapy patients often get sick right after treatment, because their immune system cannot fight anymore. For a chemotherapy patient, a cold is not just a cold. A cold could quickly turn into pneumonia.

Chemotherapy and radiation are applicable when the cancer is localized, meaning there is a target. Typically, chemotherapy is offered to stage 2 and stage 3 patients, when the cancer has not metastasized. Interestingly, there are more people dying from stage 2 and stage 3 cancer than stage 4.

I think of my diagnosis as a blessing because I had no isolated tumors for chemotherapy to target. The tumors in

---

4   Winters, Nasha, and Jess Higgins Kelley. *The Metabolic Approach to Cancer: Integrating Deep Nutrition, the Ketogenic Diet, and Nontoxic Bio-Individualized Therapies.* White River Junction, VT: Chelsea Green Publishing, 2017.

my upper body were in three areas: chest, abdomen and pelvis, and lymph nodes in the right armpit. Basically, the target was my entire upper body.

A chemotherapy treatment typically lasts six weeks: one treatment a week, and sometimes two. Chemotherapy patients often feel nauseous, lose their appetite, and feel extremely weak. These effects can—and should—be offset by an integrative treatment therapy. **Remember, not only does integrative medicine help detox the body, but it rebuilds the immune system, too.**

THE CHRONIC FACTOR

"You can't always control what goes on outside, but you can always control what goes on inside."

—WAYNE DYER

Clearly, cancer results mostly from metabolic causes. There are simply too many people dying from cancer for us to be genetically predisposed to the disease. In the United States, approximately 40 percent of men and women will be diagnosed with cancer at some point in their lives. Cancer kills 595,690 Americans each year, or approximately 1,630 per day.[5] Any integrative doctor will tell you that we are doing this to ourselves. Our internal terrain is so damaged that it

---

5   Stengler, Mark. *Outside the Box Cancer Therapies: Alternative Therapies That Treat and Prevent Cancer.* Carlsbad, CA: Hay House, Inc., 2019.

becomes a perfect breeding ground for any chronic illness, like cancer.

In this day and age, we live in a constant "chronic" state. We have chronic worry, fear, anger, stress, inflammation, and no sleep. If everything in our lives is chronic, how would this not breed a chronic disease?

Take inflammation as an example, which is a precursor to diseases. Weight training causes inflammation, which is good for the body. However, inflammation can easily become chronic if overdone and persistent.

The bottom line is that we have forgotten how to take care of ourselves. At some point, we will pay for this. I certainly did.

There is no denying that cancer has become an everyday disease. As much as this is sad, it is also good news because it means we can take steps to heal ourselves! If cancer is metabolic, then we can use a healthy lifestyle as medicine, which is what worked for me. Medicine does not have the power to make people *want* to change to get better—we need to do that ourselves. I got rid of my tumors by changing the way I live from A to Z!

LIFESTYLE AS MEDICINE

"He who takes medicine and neglects to diet wastes the skill of his doctors."

—CHINESE PROVERB

If our lifestyles are causing cancer, the key to beating cancer is within those lifestyles. We need natural medicine and approaches that treat underlying issues, not only drugs that treat our symptoms on a surface level.

In treating cancer through lifestyle, your medicine is your **food**. Your medicine is your **positive and empowering thoughts**. Your medicine is your **quiet time, lack of stress, and ability to forgive yourself**. Your medicine is joy! With this approach, you send your body the right messages for it to avoid illness and thrive.

Alternative medicine treats the body holistically, which includes scrutinizing your diet. If you lean into the belief that cancer is metabolic, you realize that nutrition is a powerful force for healing.

JOURNAL EXERCISE: EVALUATE YOUR LIFESTYLE

Many of us experience chronic inflammation, anxiety, depression, and other ailments—all of which can contribute to or exacerbate more serious illnesses. To heal, you must identify the lifestyle sources of your chronic problems.

Think about all the things we do in our lives that make us sick and answer the following questions:

What do you do in your life that promotes wellness?

How often do you practice solitude and meditation?

How often do you replace "react" with "respond" by taking deep breaths?

How often do you practice self-love and compassion?

How often do you *feel* gratitude? Thinking gratitude is not the same as actually feeling it. Make sure your gratitude is genuine.

Have you created healthy boundaries to protect your well-being?

Give your lifestyle an honest evaluation and list everything you do that hurts you and everything that makes you healthier.

Chapter 6

DIET AND NUTRITION

THE HEALING POWER OF FOOD

"Let food by thy medicine and medicine be thy food."

—HIPPOCRATES

Eating a healthy diet and meeting your nutritional requirements are necessary parts of any cancer treatment plan—both as a method to heal your body and to keep you strong. In fact, this is not only relevant to people with a cancer diagnosis; we should all be committed to living with these practices. If you don't have cancer, clean eating and good nutrition can still improve your health and provide preventative benefits.

After my diagnosis, it did not take long for me to see the effects of the cancer draining the nutrients and calories from my body. In less than a week after being diagnosed, my body weight dropped from 111 pounds to 89 pounds! I lost muscle mass and fat, which made the skin on my arms and legs hang down because there wasn't enough left to hold it up. My body shrunk to pure skin and bones.

I had always been proud of my full figure, but now, all I saw when I looked in the mirror was an extra layer of wrinkled skin. My abdomen had turned concave, almost like I had a hole in the middle of my body. I went from looking like a strong and competitive tennis athlete with muscular legs and defined shoulders to a frail-looking body that at any given moment would be blown away by the wind. Most of the clothes I had were fitted but they hung on my weak, thin body. It was hard to see myself like this every day.

NUTRITIONAL THERAPY IS A MUST

"The doctor of the future will no longer treat the human frame with drugs, but rather will cure and prevent disease with nutrition."

—THOMAS EDISON

As a chef, it was only natural that I immediately turned to food as medicine. When I realized I needed to heal with food, I had one of the first "ah-ha!" moments I would experience throughout my journey. Now, I understood why I studied to become a chef! I had to learn to use food to help me get healthier and thrive again. As we all know, for thousands of years, herbs and spices have been used as medicines. I could use food as medicine, too. I knew I needed to create a healthy and strict diet that nourished my body so I would not continue to lose weight.

I knew what diet was best for me, but not everyone agreed. My daughter Karina joined me at an appointment with my Western oncologist. She expressed concerns that I had eliminated carbohydrates, sugar, dairy, and all animal protein from my diet. She made her point and asked, "How are you supposed to gain weight when you've imposed such a restrictive diet on yourself?"

My oncologist responded by reassuring me that there was nothing wrong with my diet. I had a healthy diet and I should not change it because it was important for me to gain weight. I had to eat what I wanted to avoid cachexia. According to Dr. Nasha Winters and Jess Higgins Kelley, "Cachexia is when cancer patients experience 'wasting from within,' a syndrome that is responsible for eventually killing an estimated 50–80 percent of patients."[6]

---

6   Winters, Nasha, and Jess Higgins Kelley. *The Metabolic Approach to Cancer: Integrating Deep Nutrition, the Ketogenic Diet, and Nontoxic Bio-Individualized Therapies.* White River Junction, VT: Chelsea Green Publishing, 2017.

DEFINING A HEALING DIET

"To keep the body in good health is a duty, otherwise we shall not be able to keep our mind strong and clear."

—THE BUDDHA

At this point in my treatment, I had limited energy to spend every day, so I made a conscious decision to channel the energy I did have into healing myself. I chose not to waste any time convincing anyone of my methods. **I relied on intuition—if my actions felt right, that was enough for me.** As I continued to lose weight every day, I understood the urgency to gain at least some of it back again. However, I needed to gain healthy weight. Based on the research I had done, this meant a clean diet without any added toxins, carbohydrates, sugar, dairy, or animal protein.

I understand why a lot of people would find these dietary changes difficult to make. But I committed to the restrictions because my actions aligned with my mind. My wish to live was so extreme that I needed to take equally extreme actions to get rid of the tumors in my body and prevent the cancer cells from growing.

Only later in my journey, and after reading a book by Dr. Thomas Seyfried from Yale University and Boston College on how the ketogenic diet is the ideal diet for most cancer patients, did I realize that I was following a modified version of a ketogenic diet. A ketogenic diet consists of low carbohydrates, a small amount of protein, and a large amount of healthy fat and vegetables. The only difference between a ketogenic diet and my diet was that I ate no animal protein. I made this change because my body was already acidic and eating meat would have made it worse.

DOCTOR'S VOICE: TREATING CANCER WITH NUTRITION

"I worked with Veronica on enhancing her nutrition by adding back clean animal protein, reducing sugars and starches, and increasing even more vegetables in her diet. One of the serious side effects of lung cancer is muscle wasting or cachexia. Since she had lost so much lean body mass (she weighed 103 pounds with a BMI of 18.25) and was underweight, it was a priority to build her quickly back to a normal BMI (20-25). BMI stands for "body mass index" and is a measure of your height and weight. Fortunately, her digestion was working very well, and for the next month, she worked on getting down whey protein and greens shakes and easy-to-digest green juices. She reduced her natural sugar intake as well (fruit and honey) for blood sugar balance and continued with a light exercise regimen (stationary biking)."

Normally, the body uses glucose from carbohydrates to create energy in the body. By eliminating carbohydrates and sugar from your diet, you are forcing your body to use healthy fat for fuel instead of glucose. Why is this important? According to Dr. Thomas Seyfried, cancer cells thrive off glucose. When we remove carbohydrates from our diets, we are starving the cancer cells.[7]

Disease can make it difficult to control blood glucose levels, so it's important to manage yours with diet as much as possible. As Miriam Kalamian writes in her book *Keto for Cancer*, "I can't emphasize enough what a deleterious effect inflammation or injury has on blood glucose levels, whether caused by cancer or its treatment. The same goes for external stressors, such as poor sleep, fatigue, anxiety, or feeling overwhelmed by what's happening in your life. All of these can lead to a rise in your stress hormone levels, which in turn stimulates your liver to make new glucose."[8]

To learn more about the science behind this metabolic theory and the reason the ketogenic diet is the best for people with cancer, I recommend reading *Cancer as a Metabolic Disease* by Dr. Thomas N. Seyfried, professor of neurogenetics and neurochemistry at Yale University and Boston College.

---

7   Seyfried, Thomas N. *Cancer as a Metabolic Disease: on the Origin, Management and Prevention of Cancer.* Hoboken (New Jersey): John Wiley, 2012.

8   Kalamian, Miriam. *Keto for Cancer: Ketogenic Metabolic Therapy as a Targeted Nutritional Strategy.* White River Junction, VT: Chelsea Green Publishing, 2017.

FOOD AS MEDICINE

"The food you eat can be either the safest and most powerful form of medicine or the slowest form of poison."

—ANN WIGMORE

The best medicine for your body is eating whole and organic foods. Processed and refined food have been altered so these types of food are not considered whole foods. However, vegetables, fruits, whole grains, and legumes are examples of whole foods. Aim to eat a diet that includes plenty of green leafy vegetables, fruits as treats, legumes (mostly beans; ensure they are prepared properly to eliminate a naturally occurring, but toxic, protein called lectin), and few whole grains.

According to Dr. Steven Gundry, eating foods with lectin has a negative effect on your digestive system and causes brain fog, inflammation, and skin issues. In simple terms, lectins prevent your body from absorbing the nutrients and minerals that are in the other foods that you eat.[9]

When I eat carbohydrates, I opt for complex carbs like quinoa. At the beginning of my healing journey, I created a rule for myself that made it easy to avoid simple carbs: do not eat anything white. Later, I realized my approach might be more severe than necessary. However, I had decided to

---

9   Gundry, Steven R. *The Plant Paradox: the Hidden Dangers In "Healthy" Foods That Cause Disease And Weight Gain.* Tantor Media, Inc., 2017.

live, which meant eating foods with healing properties and avoiding foods that created acidity or chronic inflammation in my body (i.e. red meat and gluten).

My main nutrition goal was to slow down the cancer and tumor growth. When I learned sugar feeds cancer, I stopped eating sugar. If you are in the same position, **I strongly suggest you cut out sugar, too.**

HOME-COOKED MEALS

As much as possible, you want to eat whole-food, unprocessed, home-cooked meals. Dining out at restaurants is not always a good idea because of the following reasons:

1. You do not know what kind of oil the restaurant is using. Other than the oils I have listed below, all other oils I do not consider to be healthy.
   - Organic Extra Virgin Olive Oil (EVOO)
   - Organic Coconut Oil
   - Organic Avocado Oil
2. You do not know if the produce ingredients are organic.
3. You do not know if the meat protein is grass-fed and hormone and antibiotic-free.
4. You do not know if the seafood is contaminated or not.

By purchasing your own ingredients and cooking at home, you know exactly what you are putting into your body. Not sure what to cook? See **Appendix B** for healthy recipe ideas.

Was it hard for me to give up so many types of foods? Think of it this way. On my left was a chocolate soufflé, which has always been my favorite dessert. But, on my right, was my **life**.

For me, the decision was obvious.

SUGAR CONFUSION

"Sugar appears to cause pleasure with a price that is difficult to discern immediately and paid in full only years or decades later."

—GARY TAUBES

When I suggest avoiding sugar, I mean **all** sugar, which includes more than candy and pastries. To keep things simple, we can say there are two types of sugar: natural sugars, which come from fruits and vegetables, and refined sugars, which are used to sweeten foods.

Our bodies digest refined sugar faster than natural sugar. Have you ever wondered why you are still hungry after eating pastries? It is because refined sugar causes your insulin and sugar levels to spike, while fruit contains fiber, which keeps your body satiated for longer.

However, once natural and refined sugars pass through your stomach and into your intestine, your body cannot tell the difference. **As far as your body is concerned, donuts and blueberries are both made from sugar. The only difference is the calories.**

The bottom line is that there is no shortcut. If you want to live, forget about sugar entirely and ignore the cravings. After approximately two weeks without sugar, your cravings will disappear. You can do this!

PRIORITIZE YOUR IMMUNE SYSTEM

"The first wealth is health."

—RALPH WALDO EMERSON

When choosing what to eat, pick foods that will strengthen your immune system. More than any other type of food, this means eating an **abundance of green leafy vegetables.**

Remind yourself that you are fighting a battle to get rid of cancer. Think of your immune system as the soldiers fighting to keep you healthy and free from infections, bacteria, and viruses. Not only does your immune system get rid of dead cells, but cancer cells, too. **You are only as good as your immune system.**

Food rich in nutrients helps the immune system kill cancer cells. As Dr. Stephen Paget wrote in *The Lancet* in 1889, "Cancer metastasis involves a complicated biochemical

SUGAR IN DISGUISE

Beware of these sweeteners! Yes, some are low-glycemic, meaning they will not spike your blood sugar, but nonetheless, your body knows them as sugar. Let's not give the cancer cell what it needs to grow—**sugar**!

- Agave juice, nectar, and syrup
- Barbados sugar
- Barley malt or barley malt syrup
- Beet sugar
- Brown rice syrup
- Brown sugar
- Buttered syrup
- Cane sugar, juice, or syrup
- Caramel
- Carob syrup
- Castor sugar
- Coconut sugar
- Confectioners' or powdered sugar
- Corn glucose syrup
- Corn sweetener or syrup
- Date sugar
- Dextrin and dextrose
- Dried raisin sweetener
- Fructose
- Fruit juice
- Golden syrup
- Granular sweetener or sugar
- High-fructose corn syrup
- Honey
- Lactose
- Malt sweetener or syrup
- Molasses
- Raw sugar
- Refiner's syrup
- Rice syrup
- Saccharose
- Sorghum
- Starch sweetener
- Sucrose
- Sugar
- Turbinado sugar

'conversation' between the seed and the soil."[10] In this case, cancer is the seed and the human body is the soil.

Clearly, something went wrong with my immune system, which is the reason I got cancer. Now that I look back at my life with more awareness, I believe my immune system suffered from the intense stress, devastation, and despair I felt after I started my divorce process in December 2015. What I thought would be an amicable divorce turned out to be a betrayal beyond what I ever could have imagined.

THE DIVORCE DIET: EATING MYSELF TO ILLNESS

"We are what we eat…and think, and breathe, and do."

—PATRICK QUILLIN, PHD, RD, CNS

From a holistic point of view, many of my problems, including my poor diet, stemmed from the emotional turmoil of my divorce. According to Norman Cousins's book *Anatomy of an Illness*, "emotional stress can weaken the immune system and can make an individual susceptible to infections and cancer."[11] My cancer story would be incomplete without mentioning my divorce because I believe it set the illness in motion.

---

10 Paget, Stephen. "The Distribution Of Secondary Growths In Cancer Of The Breast." *The Lancet* 133, no. 3421 (1889): 571–73. https://doi.org/10.1016/s0140-6736(00)49915-0.

11 Cousins, Norman, and Dubos René Jules. *Anatomy of an Illness as Perceived by the Patient: Reflections on Healing and Regeneration.* Toronto: Bantam Books, 1985.

In hindsight, I should have divorced the father of my children over a decade earlier than I did. However, I was raised to believe that a mother should take care of everyone in her family first. In doing so, I cheated myself out of the self-love that I have always deserved.

I waited until my son started college in fall 2015 to divorce my husband. In hindsight, this has to be the biggest mistake I have ever made in my entire life. As I mentioned earlier in the book, my ex-husband had already been gathering all kinds of evidence such as old texts and emails documenting when and with whom I spent time and joined on vacation. He had printouts of text exchanges between us for over a decade. I didn't even know you could print texts from your phone!

I was naïve to believe him when we agreed that we would have an amicable divorce. I never doubted him because I thought he could never hurt me. I am the mother of his three children, and hurting me is hurting our children, which I could never do. Sadly, this was not the case. The divorce was as far from amicable as it could possibly be. In fact, he was incredibly smart in knowing exactly how to hurt me. The mindset of devastation, despair, and hopelessness I felt during this time is what caused my immune system to collapse and cancer to take root in my body. I allowed my ex-husband and the divorce to almost kill me, and as soon as I realized this, I made sure I did everything to take back my power and stay alive! Enough playing a victim.

Your mindset matters, especially when it comes to food. Your food affects your mood, and, in turn, your mood affects your eating decisions. During my divorce, I developed awful eating habits and did not sleep. I had no time because I was scrambling to gather information for my divorce, nor did I have any appetite. I would go days without eating, drinking, and sleeping. When I did eat, I turned to Tootsie Rolls as my one comfort food.

Remember, your food can either make you healthy and thriving, or it can kill you. Saving your life means making the right choices: what you think, what words you use, what you eat and drink—it all matters.

A DIET RESET

"Thou shouldst eat to live; not live to eat."

—SOCRATES

I woke up one day and thought, *I have to reset my body.* My internal terrain resembled a fish tank filled with dirty water. I would take credit for this realization, but I know now it was the guidance I needed from God and the universe.

By chance, I met Karen, who would later prepare a staple of

GUIDANCE FROM GUARDIAN ANGELS

When you ask, you receive. God sent me two angels: Maara and Karen. Maara was a friend in my indoor cycling class who insisted I see Karen. Despite being weak and tired, I asked one of my best friends, Emily, to come with me to talk to this woman. I remember the first thing Karen told me: "You're not going to die. You don't have death in your eyes."

I cried like a baby. You can't imagine how powerful it was to hear these words even though I did not know the person saying it to me. All I had heard before that moment was that I was going to die because I had an "incurable" cancer. But this woman gave me so much hope with what she said to me, and I wanted so much to believe her. To me, she was God's messenger reassuring me that I would be fine, but it would be a journey before I was healed.

Karen was incredibly generous with her time and advice on what I needed to do to jumpstart healing my body naturally. This was another test of my truth: I will not leave any stone unturned. Karen told me to do things I thought I would never try, but when you want to live and someone is in front of you telling you what to do to stay alive, YOU DO IT!

After all, what is there to lose? You have already been told that your disease is "incurable." This was the beginning of me listening to my heart and gut. The beginning of pushing through my fear of the unknown. My first leap of faith.

Everything Karen told me was said with so much conviction, so much passion, so much positive energy, and with so much certainty that it was hard to not do everything she told me to do. Karen talked to me about the importance of having my body pH balanced, drinking green juices, and finally, the big one, taking high doses of cannabis Rick Simpson oil (RSO), which I will discuss in the next chapter and include in my treatment protocol.

my healing diet, fresh green juice (juice made from organic fresh vegetables and low-sugar fruits and vegetables), when I grew too weak to prepare it myself. Around this time, I also learned about the alkaline diet, which would help decrease the high acidity in my body. As I described earlier, having an acidic body weakens the immune system and allows disease to develop.

Certain foods make our bodies acidic, including processed, fried, and junk foods. Without even knowing it, we regularly consume foods that poison us. When I learned eating meat can create an acidic body, I eliminated meat from my diet. Eating whole, organic foods helped reinstate my body to its normal pH level.

As much as possible, eat organic food. I know organic food is expensive, which is why I have included a list of the Dirty Dozen, which are foods that are highly contaminated, as well as the Clean Fifteen, which are foods that are less likely to have contaminates. See **Appendix C** for lists of other high-quality foods you should work into your diet.

If you can't afford organic, shop at farmer's markets and know the local farm you are buying from. You can ask whether their farming practices are pesticide and herbicide free or not. The same is true for your animal protein. Make sure you know that the animals are not full of antibiotics and hormones, which are used to make them gain weight faster.

WHEN SHOULD YOU BUY ORGANIC?

Making the right food choices is not just about whether to pick a fruit over a donut, but also making sure that you know where and how your food is being grown. It is important to source the highest-quality foods, preferably organic produce from your local farmers.

If you need to be selective about buying organic because of higher prices, choose the foods on the Dirty Dozen list. You will benefit more from purchasing those fruits and vegetables grown organically. With foods on the Clean Fifteen list, you can get away with buying non-organic because they tend to be less contaminated.

THE DIRTY DOZEN

According to the US Department of Agriculture, the Dirty Dozen are vegetables and fruits that have the highest levels of pesticides. As much as possible, only buy organic:

- Apples
- Celery
- Cherries
- Grapes
- Kale
- Nectarines
- Peaches
- Pears
- Potatoes
- Spinach
- Strawberries
- Tomatoes

THE CLEAN FIFTEEN

The Clean Fifteen are foods that are less likely to have pesticides, so do not worry too much if you can't find organic:

- Asparagus
- Avocado
- Broccoli
- Cabbage
- Cantaloupes
- Cauliflower
- Eggplant
- Honeydew
- Kiwis
- Mushrooms
- Onions
- Papayas
- Pineapples
- Sweet corn
- Sweet peas

Whether you're eating plants or animals, it is important to be aware that whatever is sprayed on these plants, and whatever has been fed to the animals, you are ingesting as well. Herbicides, pesticides, antibiotics, and hormones are toxins in your body.

IDENTIFY HIDDEN TOXINS

"By cleansing your body on a regular basis and eliminating toxins from your environment, your body can begin to heal itself, prevent disease, and become more strong and resilient than you ever thought possible! I firmly believe the definition of a doctor should be one who teaches, not one who prescribes."

—DR. EDWARD GROUP III

Along with eating organic, whole, high-quality foods, you also need to identify any hidden toxins in your diet. Many types of fish (especially tuna), for example, are high in heavy metals and should be avoided.

Animals raised on factory farms are a source of another hidden pollutant: antibiotics. When those animals get slaughtered and sold as meat, the antibiotics fed to them enter our bloodstream and can kill beneficial gut bacteria and interfere with our natural immune systems. I made the decision to give up meat altogether, but if you do choose to eat meat, please take the time to make sure it is grass-fed, which typically indicates higher quality, and antibiotic free.

Similarly, you want to be sure any oils or sauces you are cooking with do not contain impurities or toxins.

SUPPLEMENT YOUR DIET: LIFE CHANGING

"Health is not valued till sickness comes."

—THOMAS FULLER

If you are not already taking supplements, let me ask you a quick question: why not?

Nowadays, it is unrealistic to believe that you can get every nutrient you need from food alone. Unfortunately, our soil has been compromised due to pesticides and over-farming.

COOKING WITH OLIVE OIL

Olive oil has so many health benefits, but you must educate yourself on which one to buy and for what usage. Some of the benefits of olive oil include:

- High in monounsaturated fat and contains oleic acid, which helps with cardiovascular disease.
- Rich in antioxidants that help with disease prevention.
- Known to help with cognition function. Studies have shown that it helps with Alzheimer's disease.
- Helps with inflammation, including pain from arthritis.
- Nourishing for your skin and hair.

You want to only buy olive oil with the lowest level of free fatty acids and high amounts of polyphenols. When choosing an olive oil, consider the following differences:

- Extra Virgin Olive Oil (EVOO): Highest quality, best flavor, and fragrant. EVOO has the least free fatty-acid content. "Extra Virgin" means no solvents or chemicals were used to extract the oil from the olives. EVOO is my preferred oil for all cooking.
- Virgin Olive Oil: Satisfactory flavor with a slightly higher free fatty-acid content than an EVOO.
- U.S. Olive Oil: This is an oil mix of both virgin and refined oils. **I do not recommend this.**
- U.S. Refined Olive Oil: This is an oil made from refined oils with some restrictions on the processing. **I do not recommend this.**

I use EVOO for all types of meal preparations, including salads, sauces, sautéing, and baking. It enhances the flavor of your dishes. Keep in mind that in Europe, it is not unusual to fry using olive oils. However, I do not do this. Olive oil has a low smoke point, which means that if it is exposed to high heat, it will create toxic smoke.

"Extra" virgin or just plain "virgin"?

If you want to enjoy the maximum health benefits of olive oil, purchase the highest quality: extra virgin olive oil.

Extra virgin oil is pure, cold-pressed olives. Be sure to check if blends were used even when it says cold pressed. Sometimes they combine cold-pressed olive oil with processed oils. The oil in this case has a lighter color with a more neutral flavor.

Does the color of the olive oil matter?

The color I like to buy is either deep green to bright yellow. The more color, the more chlorophyll and polyphenols.

I suggest you purchase only olive oil in dark bottles. You need to protect it from the light, heat, and oxidation. This helps retain its nutrient levels.

Unlike wine, olive oil has a short shelf life. It should be stored in the dark and away from the heat. Do not store the bottle behind your stove. Like food, buy olive oil fresh whenever possible.

Ever since agriculture became a mass-production endeavor, the quality of the food we eat has decreased. The food we eat today is simply not as nutrient dense as it was many years ago.

By taking supplements, you get nutrients you would not necessarily get from food alone. For example, it is no secret that *everyone* is deficient in vitamin D, no matter how healthy you are. We need vitamin D to fight off infections, regulate inflammation, and maintain normal cell growth. For that reason, vitamin D should be taken by everyone. But did you know that taking vitamin D alone is not good enough? You have to take vitamin K with it to improve absorption and to protect your body from the risk of toxicity.

Your doctor will know exactly which supplements to recommend for you. To know if these supplements are being absorbed by and assimilated into your body, you should also ask your doctor for a nutritional test.

There are several reasons to take supplements:

1. Supplements can be viewed as an add-on to the standard modern food intake, which is deprived of nutrients.
2. Supplements can help eliminate toxins in your body.
3. Certain supplements have anticancer properties.
4. Supplements boost the immune system.

Your doctor will also recommend reputable brands and speak about dosages with you. While I offer brief descriptions about the supplements I have taken, I encourage you to do your own research and ask your doctor for complete information on the benefits of each supplement. It is crucial to purchase good quality supplements, as others have fillers.

Many supplements have anticancer properties. Cancer fighting supplements are essential to any comprehensive cancer treatment strategy; they attack cancer cells which constantly try to outsmart your treatment protocol. Additionally, they help to eliminate circulating tumor cells (CTC), which travel through your body and promote metastasis.

Curcumin is a powerful anti-inflammatory which is used for cancer treatment by naturopathic doctors. This is the main ingredient in turmeric, a version of Indian saffron. Although there is no actual evidence that curcumin prevents cancer, integrative medicine believes it kills cancer cells and prevents further advancement of tumors.

Oral vitamin C has a different effect on the body than intravenous high dose vitamin C (IVC); the former is essentially a milder version. My naturopathic doctor believes IVC eradicates cancer, shrinks tumors, and stops the disease from metastasizing. You could never match the dosage of intravenous vitamin C with oral vitamin C. However, an oral vitamin C supplement boosts the immune system and acts as a powerful antioxidant. Take care when choosing vitamin C supplements. Ask your doctor for recommendations; you are looking for a supplement which is bioavailable to the body and **not** made with genetically modified corn. Keep in mind that vitamin C can also be found in foods like broccoli.

Vitamin D3 is another important supplement which is critical in our immune defense to fight off serious infections and cancer. It also helps reduce inflammation and mold healthy cells. However, certain fat-soluble vitamins need fat or oil for the body to absorb them. Unless you are taking a vitamin D3 supplement encapsulated with oil or eating it with an avocado or nut butter, your body is not digesting the vitamin. I try to buy gel caps instead of tablets, because the gel cap vitamins are packaged in oil for best absorption. Most people are deficient in vitamin D3, no matter how much sun we are exposed to. I usually take 5,000 micrograms per day, but I recommend asking your doctor to test your vitamin D3 to determine an appropriate dosage for you.

Everyone should be taking **probiotics**: live microorganisms which balance your gut bacteria. Our bodies are imbalanced when the bad bacteria outweigh the good, which can happen when eating an unhealthy diet or taking antibiotics. Make sure you take probiotics at night before bed. Additionally, you might consider rotating the brands you buy so your body does not get used to one strain.

Our bodies do not produce **zinc**. Unless you are getting enough zinc from your diet (which you are probably not), it is important to take a zinc supplement to boost immune function, cell growth and division. If you have cancer, cell growth is key for your body to grow healthy cells.

Just because you eat a nutritional diet, that does not mean your body is absorbing the nutrients and vitamins or digesting them properly. This is where it is helpful to take **digestive enzymes** to help break down the food you eat so it can flow more easily through your system. Enzymes are key to digesting the fats, protein, and carbohydrates in your food. Unlike other supplements, enzymes are taken **before** eating.

Omega-3s are essential fatty acids (EFAs). Found in fatty fish, they offer many health benefits such as preventing inflammation, lowering high blood pressure, preventing mental deterioration, combating depression, and most importantly, preventing the spread of cancer cells!

Melatonin is a powerful antioxidant; it is the hormone produced by the pineal gland in our brain at night. Unfortunately, the artificial lights from our phones, TVs, and computer screens cause our bodies to produce less melatonin. A low dose of melatonin can help with insomnia. When you take a higher dose, melatonin becomes an antioxidant which inhibits tumor growth and metastasis. Again, determine your dosage with the help of a health professional.

Magnesium is another mineral which is not produced by the body, meaning we can only get it from our diets or supplements. Without magnesium, your body will struggle to build proteins into a production of energy. I take magnesium right before I go to bed.

Chlorella is a type of freshwater algae that inhibits the absorption of heavy metals in the body, especially mercury. These days, chlorella is considered a superfood. It is very nutritious, as it contains proteins, vitamins, minerals, antioxidants, and omega-3 fats. In addition, chlorella is supposed to boost the immune system to battle against bacteria and viruses, as well as fight cancer and other diseases. Personally, I take chlorella supplements to make sure my body is constantly detoxing from toxins, especially heavy metals.

Disclaimer: In this book, I am sharing *my* personal experience with supplements. Although most supplements are safe, I still encourage you to talk to a health professional about designing a supplement list for *you*. This should happen after you have completed nutritional tests to evaluate what nutrients your body needs, as well as your levels of absorption and detoxification. In my case, we used the NutrEval test by Genova Diagnostics.

BALANCE YOUR HORMONES

"Stress is the most powerful carcinogen imaginable. It increases inflammation, spikes blood sugar, and disables the immune system. Metastasis is promoted when the body or mind is stressed."

—DR. NASHA WINTERS

When you feel stressed, you release hormones that create dysfunction in your body—including how your body processes food. You cannot properly use the nutrients you eat if your hormones are imbalanced.

Around the time of my divorce, I spent years living in extreme stress. I found out later that I had been overproducing certain hormones, including the stress hormone, cortisol. This is what we call **chronic stress**; I effectively lived in fight or flight mode. The stress never left my body.

Modern society suffers from an epidemic of stress. Our bodies typically respond to stress by creating an imbalance in our hormones. As the stress hormone increases, blood glucose increases, too, which triggers a cascade of other health problems. For example, you cannot lose weight while your body is in fight or flight mode because it cannot use fat for fuel, only glucose.

Some of my clients are frustrated about their inability to lose weight. While their bodies are mostly thin, they have a layer of visceral fat around their waistlines or their lower back. To me, that fat points to gut issues and stored fat because of stress, a precursor for any chronic disease. If you have a similar layer of stubborn fat, you might have a hormone imbalance.

To detect hormone imbalances, you can take a **cortisol**

stress hormone test, which measures the cortisol in your saliva three times a day. You spit first thing in the morning, at midday, and right before you go to sleep. In theory, your cortisol level should be elevated in the morning, slightly more elevated by midday, and lowest before you go to bed, when you should be calmest. In my case, my cortisol levels were ridiculously high at night. Little did I know how much my stress took a toll on my insides; I never made the connection between mind, body, and spirit before being diagnosed with cancer.

BODILY FUNCTIONS KEEP US BALANCED

"The natural healing force within each of us is the greatest force in getting well."

—HIPPOCRATES

In addition to stress-induced hormone imbalances, which interfere with nutrient absorption, another problem many— if not most—people suffer from is dysfunctional digestion. **Health starts in the gut.** If you are not properly digesting your food, you are not absorbing the necessary nutrients, nor are you eliminating the toxins harming your body.

In a normally functioning body, three bodily functions occur daily: urination, defecation, and perspiration. Why? Through these processes, toxins leave the body. When these things are not happening, your body retains toxins. In other words, you are poisoning yourself.

This dysfunction starts a chain reaction where other organs, including your liver and kidneys, become compromised because you have not eliminated the toxins from inside your body.

When I first did an infrared sauna treatment (a light-based therapy used to treat pain and promote detoxification) I sweated out everything I had inside of me. Instantly, I could tell my body hadn't been properly processing and eliminating the toxins in my food because when I wiped my skin, the towel came away black. My doctor explained that was my body's way of detoxing. Everything that had been trapped in my body was *finally* getting a chance to be released. Now, when I wipe my skin after such a treatment, the towel is clear, as it should be.

Bodily functions are crucial to good health and should not be taboo. For some reason, nobody likes to talk about these **natural** processes. However, the less we talk about these topics, the more people won't recognize signs of imbalance and will suffer because of it. Instead of being an embarrassment, every trip to the bathroom should be a celebration because it is an opportunity to remove toxins from your body. Yes, including cancer cells!

To get an idea of the way things are working (or not) in your gut, ask your doctor for a gut microbial test.

We need to stop using our bodies as garbage trucks. We are not built to store anything bad inside of us, and when that happens, we only breed disease.

A nutrient-rich diet, balanced hormones, and good bodily functions are the secrets to a healthy life for anyone, not just for those battling cancer. Over the last few years, I have helped my friends, family, and clients implement these strategies into their daily routines. A cortisol saliva test and vitamin C and D supplements can benefit **anyone**.

HOW FOOD TRIGGERS DISEASE

"When diet is wrong, medicine is of no use. When diet is correct, medicine is of no need."

—ANCIENT AYURVEDIC PROVERB

Cancer cells will only be triggered if they are given fuel in the form of sugar. In my case, my divorce caused me to increase my sugar intake dramatically; it is difficult to imagine how many Tootsie Rolls I ate during that period of my life. The more sugar I ate, the more I craved. Not only was the sugar intake addictive, but it triggered the cancer cells in my body. The common denominator in many diseases, such as diabetes, which is a precursor for cancer, is sugar.

Every living person has cancer cells in their body. Usually, the cells are harmlessly removed. The dangerous part is when those cells get triggered and create disease.

Even before an unhealthy diet triggers disease, nutrient-poor food makes us feel sick and lethargic. The reason you suddenly feel tired at three o'clock in the afternoon is because you ate something full of sugar at lunchtime, which spiked your insulin levels but made your energy crash shortly afterward.

The fact that so many kids get diagnosed with ADHD can be attributed to the poor quality of their food. Macaroni and cheese and hamburgers do nothing good for our internal systems. Unfortunately, we have accepted a bad diet as unavoidable, but as far as our bodies are concerned, it is **not** the norm.

Now that I eat well, I do not feel tired throughout the day. I feel energized up until the moment I go to bed. Even after I work out, I have more energy to burn. By adopting a nutrient-rich diet and eliminating sugar, you can feel boundless energy, too.

WHAT *SHOULD* YOU EAT? REAL WHOLE FOOD

"The act of putting into your mouth what the earth has grown is perhaps your most direct interaction with the earth."

—FRANCES MOORE LAPPÉ

A good diet means getting all your vitamins. It consists of whole, organic foods, including **lots of leafy greens.**

Do yourself a favor and buy the highest-quality and cleanest foods whenever you can. See **Appendix D** for information on the shelf life of produce in your refrigerator so you can eat fruits and vegetables while they are fresh. Learn to read food labels; sugars, additives, flavor enhancers, and bad fats are usually well disguised behind unrecognizable names. Stay away from buying anything with nitrates (these are typically found in cold meats to prolong their shelf life and add food coloring).

Eat organic food as much as possible, provided you can afford it. I recommend shopping at farmers' markets because you can get higher-quality produce for lower prices. Get to know the local farm you are buying from and make sure their farming practices are free of pesticides and herbicides.

Approach the animal protein you eat with the same due diligence. If you eat animal protein, you should make sure the animals have not been injected with antibiotics or hormones to make them gain weight faster. Regardless of whether you are eating plants or animals, be aware that whatever has been sprayed or fed to them will, in turn, enter your body. All herbicides, pesticides, antibiotics, and hormones are toxic to your body.

Remember, you are only as good as your immune system. Your body is a strong, intelligent machine that can handle getting sick and healing itself, provided you have a strong immune system. According to Kris Carr in *Crazy Sexy Diet*, "If you don't think your anxiety, depression, sadness, and stress impact your health, think again. All of these emotions trigger chemical reactions in your body, which can lead to inflammation and a weakened immune system."[12]

Clearly, something went wrong with my immune system, which is why I got sick in the first place. I believe this was a result of the immense stress, devastation, and despair my poor body experienced. Now, I know better.

---

12   Carr, Kris. *Crazy Sexy Diet: Eat Your Veggies, Ignite Your Spark, and Live like You Mean It!* Guilford, Ct: Skirt, 2011.

THE POWER OF THE IMMUNE SYSTEM

"Think of the immune system like the military, there are different branches that each serve a unique function in protecting the body."

—DAT TRAN, MD

To eradicate the cancer in your body, you need a strong immune system, which does not align with a bad diet, stress, or toxins. Dr. Patrick Quillin said on this subject, "Your immune system consists of twenty trillion specialized warrior cells that are responsible for killing lethal invaders, such as cancer, yeast, bacteria, and virus. Breakdown in the immune system is at least partly responsible for cancer taking over a human body."[13]

Suppressed emotions lead to a suppressed immune system, which impairs your ability to fight infections from fungi and bacteria. Dr. Quillin explains, "In 1999, researchers at the Mayo Clinic found that 96 percent of all sinus infections were caused by fungi. Essentially, fungi enter the body through the sinus cavities creating infection, which spreads throughout the body, resulting in pain, fatigue, and eventually, cancer."[14]

Before being diagnosed with cancer, I took antibiotics

---

13   Quillin, Patrick, and Noreen Quillin. *Beating Cancer with Nutrition*. Tulsa, OK: Nutrition Times Press, 2005.

14   Ibid.

nearly every month to treat alternating infections. The doctors only cared about treating my symptoms, but nobody realized that my body had become resistant to the medicine. Although antibiotics kill bad bacteria, they also kill good bacteria in the digestive tract. The rule for most medications is that their side effects create even more toxicity in the body. This is where detoxification becomes important. How can your immune system do its job when your body is burdened with toxins?

DETOXIFYING YOUR BODY

"Food can be a poison or a cure. Why would you choose to ingest toxins when you could be taking the world's best detox medicine?"

—WOODSON MERRELL

As I have learned firsthand, under the right conditions, cancer growth can be both slowed and reversed—and I am far from the only person to experience this turn of events. According to the National Cancer Institute, there are 7 million Americans alive today who have lived five or more years after their cancer diagnosis. The lesson here is that **cancer is reversible.**

"If toxins caused the problem, then detoxification is the solution," Dr. Patrick Quillin says.[15]

---

15   Ibid.

If detoxification is key to healing, then where are the toxins coming from? Toxins are everywhere. They enter your body from medications, synthetic hormones, non-organic food contaminated with pesticides, processed food, the environment, and a toxic mind!

Follow these tips to reduce toxins in your diet and body:

- Be careful drinking tap water, as it could contain chemicals and pollutants. To improve the quality of your tap water, you can install an alkalinizing/ionized water filter at home.
- Avoid alcohol, soda, and processed foods.
- Eat baked, sautéed, and steamed foods instead of fried foods.
- Not only are fresh green juices a great source of nutrients to the body, but they provide a huge dose of enzymes and reduce inflammation, which contributes to boosting your immune system and increasing your energy. Avoid adding apples to your green juices, as they contain too much sugar.

ELIMINATE HEAVY METALS

Get proactive about removing the toxins from your body. The most damaging toxins linked to cancer are heavy metals like mercury, lead, cadmium, and aluminum. Mercury is *everywhere*. It is in the fish we eat, especially tuna. If you cannot live without fish, stick to fish with lower levels of mercury, like sardines, salmon, tilapia, North Atlantic chub mackerel, and freshwater trout.

Mercury can also be found in dental amalgams, which is a mixture used for fillings. In order to heal, your mouth needs to be clear of toxins, too. When I had all the mercury removed from my mouth, I learned I may have had an infection caused by root canals. To avoid taking any chances, I switched over to a biological dentist, which is essentially a holistic dentist that avoids harmful chemicals.

CARE FOR YOUR LYMPHATIC SYSTEM

If you did not know, our blood delivers nutrients to our cells while our lymphatic system removes the toxins. If the lymphatic system gets blocked, it cannot flush out the toxic debris, which leads to a compromised immune system. As I have mentioned, a compromised immune system is the perfect environment for disease to breed in the body. To prevent your lymphatic system from becoming blocked, add exercise, massages, dry brushing (exfoliating by rubbing a dry loofah or brush over the skin), raw foods, herbs, and plenty of lemon water to your daily routine.

TAKE TOXIN-BINDING SUPPLEMENTS

Another way to remove toxins from your body is by

taking toxin-binding supplements. I take **chlorella** daily, which cleans toxins from the food I eat and stimulates my immune system to aid faster healing.

Even if you do not have cancer, detoxification therapy should be a part of your life. During my fight with cancer, I made every effort to clear my body of toxins and reduce inflammation. I noticed the effects immediately: my bloating disappeared, I had more energy, my mind cleared, and I slept better.

The more you make detoxification a part of your daily life, the better you will equip yourself to prevent cancer and other diseases. As an added bonus, you will feel stronger and healthier.

MAKE LASTING CHANGES TO YOUR DIET

"Take care of your body. It's the only place you have to live."
—JIM ROHN

This might sound harsh but, when you are ill, you cannot cheat yourself of proper nutrition. A good diet is non-negotiable. Making long-lasting changes may be hard at first, but as soon as you start noticing positive results, eating well will become easier.

The food you eat can either help you thrive or poison you.

If you are serious about saving your life, you need to make the right choices. You are not just eating for calories anymore. **You are eating to heal yourself and to strengthen your immune system.**

Even though you may have received a prognosis predicting an end to your life, this is actually the beginning of you living in a different way. As of this moment, you are living a conscious life. Every action you take should be deliberate because its purpose is to lead you in the direction of healing.

The more you implement these practices into your daily routine, the more they will feel like a default. I changed my habits when I learned my diagnosis, but today, I continue to live this way. Whenever I put food in my mouth, I know exactly how it is benefiting my body.

Following a diagnosis, a patient probably needs more than nutrients alone to reverse the disease. In my case, with stage 4 metastasized cancer, it was unrealistic to expect that changing my diet was the only thing I needed to do to get better. Fortunately, I found holistic treatments to supercharge my healing.

JOURNAL EXERCISE: FOOD DIARY

I encourage you to write a food diary to keep track of what you eat every day. Evaluate your choices. Which foods heal your body? Which foods offer nothing but empty calories?

By noticing your unhealthy dietary habits, you can take steps to break and eliminate them. Remember, now is the time to stay active. Be conscious about the choices you are making. Now is not the time to relinquish control over your life. Now is **not** the time to give up.

Buying your food from the farmers' market instead of the supermarket is a conscious choice. You should feel excited to buy good food that will nourish your body. Appreciate the little things you do for yourself each day. Enjoy every conscious and health-focused decision you make.

———

Chapter 7

TREATMENTS

HEAL YOUR BODY

"You are the architect of your own destiny; you are the master of your own fate; you are behind the steering wheel of your life."

—BRIAN TRACY

At the time of my diagnosis, I already had extensive tumors in my upper body. They spanned my right and left sides: my right lung and chest, abdomen, pelvis, and more. Some tumors were easily measurable while others were too small and too widespread to quantify. The scan report labeled the area affected as "extensive."

From the second I learned about the tumors, I started looking for how to get rid of them. At the time, my oncologists gave me *no* hope. Instead of discussing treatments with me, the oncologists spent more time telling me the next area of metastasis—my brain! The same way they dismissed my questions about how to rid my body of this cruel and awful disease, I dismissed everything they were saying. This was the first time I felt all alone in my battle. I made it my mission to figure out what I needed to do to stay alive. I refused to give up! If there was anything I was prepared to do, it was to die trying to stay alive.

Meeting my integrative medicine doctor and beginning alternative treatments turned the tide in my mission to heal.

DOCTOR'S VOICE: HOLISTIC TREATMENTS

"Veronica was initially seen at Eisenhower Hospital's Emergency Department on September 22, 2016, for fatigue, weight loss, chest pain, lingering cough, back pain, and difficulty breathing. She was admitted to the hospital and treated for possibility of a blood clot that had moved to her lungs or a lung infection. She was put on blood thinners, antibiotics, and had a chest tube placed to drain 1600cc of fluid from around her right lung and biopsies taken.

"Through their thorough workup, she was diagnosed with metastatic non-small cell lung cancer with ALK1+ mutation on September 24, 2016. There was extensive tumor involvement of mostly her right lung (6.3 cm x 7.3 cm), with lymph node involvement throughout her chest, axilla, and upper retroperitoneum.

"Since she lived part-time in Los Angeles, Veronica transferred her care from Eisenhower to UCLA, where she was started on Alecensa (alectinib) in late November 2016 by her oncologist. Alectinib is a tyrosine kinase inhibitor drug that blocks certain proteins made by the ALK gene. Blocking these proteins may stop the growth and spread of cancer cells, especially to the brain and spinal cord. With her specific diagnosis, she was a candidate for this new targeted therapy, rather than going through chemotherapy. This treatment allowed us time to utilize all of her other naturopathic treatment protocols to help her body fight off the remaining tumors. V's treatment protocol is specific and customized to her, and it may not apply to everyone. That is the art and science of integrative oncology, and the beauty of personalized medicine.

"With her diagnosis and initial health presentation, time was of essence. Her treatment protocol had to be aggressive, and fortunately, V was a highly motivated and compliant patient. On her own, she had already changed to a vegetarian diet, started on some supplements, and cannabis "Rick Simpson oil" (RSO). I ran more blood work and a specialty lab called RGCC, which tests the efficacy of several natural therapeutics against her circulating cancer stem cells. The idea was to utilize the most effective natural therapeutic agents against her cancer cells. Note that this is a lab in Greece and is not covered by insurance.

We started her on a robust treatment protocol with direction *from her lab tests. I created monthly protocols for the next three months and rotated them every quarter. Aside from one small setback at the end of February 2017, when she developed pneumonia and was treated and resolved with antibiotics within a week, she had continued to improve leaps and bounds in her strength, vitality, and energy.*

"By June 2017, her oncologist determined that the initial large lung masses had reduced to stable micro nodules (<5mm) and stated no new disease and no evidence of disease, which continues to be evident in her most recent April 2019 scans. The side effects of the medication were minimal throughout treatment. There was no elevation of liver enzymes or bone marrow changes. There was some minimal fatigue and ankle swelling, which were resolved through exercise. Although there was never a guarantee of a cure, the outcome of her treatments has been a resounding success and a testament to her consistent hard work and dedication to living life healthfully and to the fullest!"

NO STRESS, NO DRAMA: CANNABIS OIL

I began taking Rick Simpson oil (RSO) a month after I was diagnosed. Soon enough, I built up to taking 2.5g a day! For the record, this was a lot! In my research, I read countless testimonials about RSO working for cancer patients who are still alive today. In my mind, there was no harm in doing a treatment that consisted of pure herbs. The only downside was that I often got so high I could not function. I never became addicted, but I slept for fifteen hours a day. While my mind and body needed sleep, I also needed to be awake to eat and gain weight for my oncologist.

Was I scared to try cannabis? No. I knew this was the beginning of a long healing journey, and to succeed, I had to step out of my comfort zone. The crazier the goal, the crazier the process would be.

RICK SIMPSON OIL

In 2003, a Canadian man named Rick Simpson cured his skin cancer with pure cannabis oil. Since his discovery, he has helped many people with cancer diagnoses using what is called Rick Simpson oil (RSO).

RSO is made from the Indica strain, which contains high levels of tetrahydrocannabinol, or THC. For simplicity, this is what gives the "high" associated with cannabis. Today, people talk casually about "getting high" from endorphins, the brain's feel-good chemicals produced naturally by exercise, laughing, having sex, and even from eating raw chocolate, but "getting high" from a *natural plant* seems scary and intolerable to most people! I can't help but question the motives behind why it is more normal and acceptable to take drugs like morphine than a natural plant like cannabis.

After my diagnosis, I wanted to heal holistically, and as much as I was not an advocate of drugs pre-cancer, healing with the cannabis plant was more desirable than experiencing the negative effects of the "cut, burn, and poison" approach.

For the first time in my life, I did not care what anyone thought about me, my decisions, or my treatments. I prioritized taking care of myself; that meant **no stress, no drama.** I learned to accept who I was at any given moment. The person I am now is no longer who I was a day ago.

At times, I would be stoned, weak, and always late for everything. It became a running joke among my friends that I would always be late and text a hundred times for directions. I laughed it off, and nobody ever made me feel bad. They were happy that I arrived whenever I did.

When you ask God or the universe for help, they deliver without fail. At one point, I confided in my friend Emily that I could not continue to go through my life high on cannabis. I needed to find a way to take the oil but get less stoned. One morning, I woke up and remembered my dream of making suppositories with Rick Simpson oil. I did some research and used my skills in the kitchen to make my own RSO suppositories. This was another blessing from God guiding me towards the next step in my journey. I could not have thought of those suppositories on my own; I needed God's influence to make me dream of them.

Medicine, in pill or drink form, can get into your body orally. Suppositories are another way to deliver a drug into the body without involving the stomach. When I took RSO orally, it traveled to my stomach, making me feel more stoned. Suppositories easily and rapidly absorbed into my blood, traveling to other areas of my body without affecting my mind as much. By taking suppositories, I could function somewhat normally. I would not show up to an appointment with one side of my hair not styled.

As much as cannabis helped me, I honestly did not enjoy taking it. I was usually so put together and did not like feeling slow and uncoordinated. Going through this treatment was yet another lesson in humility. It was not about how I looked or how coordinated I was; it was about believing that the RSO was shrinking the tumors that plagued my body. By thinking this way, I was reminded of my priorities. Now, my physical appearance is the least of my concerns because I have learned that during all these years when I looked amazing externally, my internal body was dirty and being poisoned!

Here, you'll learn more details about my treatment protocol as described by my integrative-medicine doctor.

DOCTOR'S VOICE: DESIGNING A TREATMENT PROTOCOL

"For simplicity, I have broken down Veronica's treatment protocol into general categories. The following information is not for diagnostic or treatment purposes. This is only to

inform the readers of options that may not be presented to them through traditional outlets.

"Also, there is a difference between retail (Amazon/Costco/ Walmart/GNC/multi-level marketing brands, etc.) and high-quality, doctor-prescribed vitamin and supplement sources/ brands. All supplements are NOT created equal, and often, you get what you pay for. Quality supplements are key for optimal health and performance. There are reasons such as bioavailability with herbs, vitamins, and minerals. Cheaper vitamins typically are made from non-bioavailable forms of the nutrients and use binders to press them into a hard-tablet, horse-pill form. Most cancer patients (and non-cancer patients) have issues with digestion and may not be able to break down and absorb these types of pills, and it is a waste of time and resources to start with poor quality supplements.

"Always ask your doctor or a healthcare professional knowl-edgeable in integrative medicine before starting any new treatment protocols. Remember that every patient's treat-ment protocol is tailored to them.

"These are the highlights of Veronica's treatments.

Intravenous (IV) therapy:

- *Multivitamin/amino acid/mineral support: In patients with a compromised immune and digestive system, in* addition to poor nutrition, they need immediate nutritional support that can bypass their gut function and infuse directly into their cells. Patients have improved quality of life with providing basic essential nutrients in the most absorbable way possible, via intravenous means.

- High-dose Intravenous Vitamin C (HDIVC): The major concept behind HDIVC and cancer is that it is used as a pro-drug for the production of hydrogen peroxide in the extracellular space, thus potentially damaging the cancer cells to stimulate apoptosis (cell death). It has been shown that some cancer cells have decreased ability to defend against the induced peroxide surge, where normal human cells can reduce the peroxide to water, thus sparing normal cells from oxidative damage. Oral dosing of vitamin C is unable to create a plasma level high enough to create any substantial peroxide formation due to its dose limiting osmotic effect on the colon. The high (25+ gram) doses of vitamin C needed to create a peroxide surge in the extracellular space required to potentially damage cancer cells can only be attained through intravenous means.

- IV Ozone and Major Auto-hemotherapy (MAH): Medical ozone is a potent regulator of the immune system by inducing leukocyte activity and the production of cytokines such as interferon gamma and beta and interleukins. It also stimulates an increase in oxygenation of tissues in plasma to create LOP (lipid oxidation products) and upregulates antioxidant enzymes and improves circulation.

- *Poly-MVA: Poly-MVA is a uniquely formulated compound containing a proprietary blend of the mineral palladium bonded to alpha-lipoic acid, vitamins B1, B2, and B12, formyl-methionine, N-acetyl cysteine, plus trace amounts of molybdenum, rhodium, and ruthenium. This formulation is designed to provide energy for compromised body systems by changing the electrical potential of human cells and facilitating aerobic metabolism within the cell. Poly-MVA may assist in boosting immune response by replenishing key nutrients and supporting cellular metabolism.*

- *Artesunate: Artesunate (ART), a derivative of artemisinin, can be a potent and selective antitumor agent as well as an antimicrobial agent. Additionally, ART appears to be a synergist with oxidative therapies such as high dose vitamin C. Artemisinin and its analogs are naturally occurring antimalarials which have shown potent anticancer activity. In primary cancer cultures and cell lines, their antitumor actions were by inhibiting cancer proliferation, metastasis, and angiogenesis. In xenograft models, exposure to artemisinin substantially reduces tumor volume and progression.*

Subcutaneous mistletoe therapy:

- *Mistletoe is one of the most common integrative oncologic therapies in Europe, especially Germany. Mistletoe is used in subcutaneous and IV preparations to support* the body through: immunomodulation through activation of macrophages, dendritic cells, and natural killer cells, enhancement of phagocytosis as well as increase of eosinophils, lymphocytes, and T-helper cells; DNA protective effects on peripheral immune cells, protection from immunosuppressive effects of chemotherapy; and antitumoral effects by induction of apoptosis and anti-angiogenesis.

Oral nutrients:

- *Genistein: Soy-derived isoflavone and phytoestrogen with antineoplastic activity. Genistein binds to and inhibits protein-tyrosine kinase, thereby disrupting signal transduction and inducing cell differentiation. It is also an EGFR, VEGF, Ras/Raf inhibitor and increases antitumor activity of gemcitabine while reducing activity of NF-kB, controlling insulin resistance.*
- *Proteolytic enzymes: downregulate MDR1/MRP (drug resistance proteins), reduce cancer resistance to chemo and other therapies.*
- *Melatonin (high dose): hormone secreted from the pineal gland in the brain, used to regulate sleep/wake cycle, melatonin significantly suppresses cell proliferation and induces apoptosis.*
- *Vitamin D3: optimal levels reduce cancer risk in multiple types of cancers.*
- *Omega-3 fish oil: anti-inflammatory, reduces cancer risk.*

- *Vascustatin: reduces angiogenesis, VEGF inhibitor.*
- *Active B vitamin complex: methylated forms of B vitamins used for energy, stress reduction, immune support.*

Herbal supplements:

- *Artemisinin: oral form of artesunate*
- *Quercetin: bioflavonoid, potent antioxidant, acts as "chemopreventor"/cancer-preventing effects, and has direct apoptotic effect on tumor cells without damaging normal cells.*
- *Agaricus Blazei: inhibits tumor growth via direct inhibition of tumor-induced angiogenesis, activates macrophages or natural killer cells and induced cytotoxic T-lymphocyte activity.*
- *Green tea extract (EGCG): antioxidant, antimicrobial, antiproliferative, pro-apoptotic via chemo-preventor effects.*
- *Curcumin: main polyphenol found in turmeric, has been shown to block NF-κB activation (anti-inflammatory) and antioxidant properties.*
- *Berberine: Berberine has been shown to exert antitumor effects through multiple routes, for example, suppressing cell proliferation, metastasis, and angiogenesis in numerous tumor types through mTOR inhibition via regulation of RARα/β and the PI3K/AKT signaling pathway."*

AM I CURED?

"It is during our darkest moments that we must focus to see the light."

—ARISTOTLE

When I share my story, people are quick to ask me if I am cured. I resist labels, so my answer is that **I am here and living my best life today.** I am more alive than I have ever been! Clearly, the six-month prognosis did not come true, but I am equally not claiming to have cured myself. All I am claiming is that my life is fulfilling and joyful after this transformation.

As people, we often seek labels for security. If there is one thing I know from this experience, one thing I learned, it's that **there is no security.** Not only has God interrupted my life plans, but he also challenged everything I believe in. He has proved me wrong in so many ways. As the Buddha says, "In the end, only three things matter: how much you loved, how gently you lived, and how gracefully you let go of things not meant for you."

According to my oncologist, I cannot claim remission because there is no cure for the type of cancer I developed. I can claim No Evidence of Disease (NED), which we saw in late 2017.

Now, it is much easier to take each day as it comes. Now, I

am happy with the fact that I am moving forward, as long as I feel better with each passing day. My focus is on the formula: the journey I took to get to where I am today. This book allows you an opportunity to follow the same formula. Stop feeling sorry for yourself and turn into the sort of person who feels excited about life, even if you have been given a short prognosis. After all, **I only found the true meaning of life when I was given a death sentence.**

Throughout your journey, revisit the core questions that will reshape your life. What kind of life are you fighting for? How do you want to transform yourself? Where is the incredible life that you are supposed to have? As you push through pain and humility, you will find the greatness of life. To make this discovery, you need to put in the inner work.

At this point in my life, I can confidently say I know who I am. Throughout this healing journey, I have picked up tools and character-building skills I would never have learned otherwise. I have taken things back to the basics, which is humbling. Three years later, I have come out stronger. I have made peace with the fact that I do not know everything, no matter how much I want to. Relinquishing control and surrendering have made living a lot easier. Magic happens when things fall into place and you let go of the illusion of control.

This book takes a naturopathic approach to healing and establishing a new lifestyle. It is not enough to change your food and try some treatments. Think of this as a permanent way of living from now on. If you want to increase your chances of staying healthy, you have to make the effort **every day**. Over time, you will get better at what you are already doing. The good news is that there are always new treatments to try. My treatment protocol has evolved over time, as should yours.

Along with treatments, you will achieve lasting good health by transforming your lifestyle.

JOURNAL EXERCISE: CREATE A CHECKLIST FOR DOCTOR APPOINTMENTS

I never discussed my natural therapies with my oncologist, but he made it clear that those treatments would not cure me. In my mind, I had no choice. At least alternative medicine gave me more hope than the Western prognosis, which said I would die in six months.

While I highly respect my oncologist, I believe his training prevents him from being open to other treatment methods. However, he has always encouraged me to do what feels right, and that is enough for me. Ultimately, he knows that I will continue to do whatever I want to do, and I am looking (and feeling) better for it. On top of that, every scan has shown the tumors shrinking or disappearing from my body.

A lesson I learned early on that will help you maintain a good relationship with your doctor is to create a checklist to take to appointments. When a patient is educated in their illness, doctors have more respect for you. They take you more seriously and involve you in the treatment process. The more you engage in your own healing journey, the more empowered you will feel about the changes you are making.

Chapter 8

LIFESTYLE

LIVE HEALTHIER EVERY DAY

"It is not a daily increase, but a daily decrease. Hack away at the inessentials."

—BRUCE LEE

If you have been sleepwalking through your life, **now is the time to wake up.**

A cancer diagnosis is the most shocking wakeup call you can get, so let your diagnosis be an opportunity to rearrange your priorities. Now, you can embrace a new lifestyle that is conducive to living a healthy life and eradicating the disease from your body.

THE DANGER OF STRESS

"Our anxiety does not come from thinking about the future, but from wanting to control it."

—KAHLIL GIBRAN

I have mentioned stress throughout this book, but in a discussion about lifestyle, it is worth reiterating because it presents such a threat to your health. Stress has become such a key part of modern life that we mistakenly believe it is normal. For many people, being stressed has become our default state. Stress has become chronic for most of us. The word "stress" means nothing anymore because we use it so loosely, when in fact, it *should* refer to a serious physiological state. Stress is silently making you sick without you even realizing it.

Where do you think your stress comes from? I came to the realization that most of my stress originates from the way I react versus respond not to *the* reality but *a* reality. Most of what is in our heads is *a* reality we made up. It is not *true* because it has not happened, and therefore, it is not *the* reality. From now on, I want you to take stress seriously. If you do feel stressed, what does that mean? What are you stressed about? Check in with yourself and ask if what is in your head is *a* reality or *the* reality.

Quite often, what we are thinking and worrying about is not true or has not happened, and yet we act like our fears are *the* reality. Ignoring stress only leads to more negative consequences. To live happy and healthy lives, we should associate ourselves with as little stress as possible. Stress is not an emotion we should be feeling every day, let alone every five minutes.

Make a conscious effort to align your words with your actions. The first step to lifestyle transformation is mindfulness. The language you use can either empower or disempower you by subtly shaping your mindset toward the positive or negative. Your words can literally make you sick, so I recommend trying to remove "stress" from your vocabulary, especially when describing your state of being. If something is making you stressed, identify what it is and **do something about it.**

Stress can also be chemical rather than mental. For example, by drinking alcohol and taking antibiotics, you are putting stress on your liver. When doctors prescribe us medicine, we take it without questioning the side effects. Be aware that there might be other options available to you other than taking antibiotics (like the alternative treatments I discussed in the previous chapter). Note, however, that you should always discuss options with your doctors and never stop taking medicine without telling them.

Medication tends to tackle the symptoms of an illness, but it does not deal with the root of the problem. If you find yourself getting sick all the time, learn about the *cause*. Stress increases your insulin, sugar, and glucose levels, which all feed cancer. The more stress you put on your body, the more difficult it will be to get rid of your tumors.

On top of everything else, stress can negatively impact your sleep, too. When people have a hard time sleeping, it is usually because their mind is too busy. Endless thoughts can cause insomnia, which is hormonal and affected by high cortisol levels, creating a vicious cycle of worry and restlessness.

WHY STRESS IS DANGEROUS FOR YOUR BODY

Stress can cause serious health consequences, especially when it is sustained over time, or chronic. Here are several effects of stress that can damage your health:

- Suppresses your immune system so it takes longer for your body to recover from illness.
- Damages your skin by causing acne.
- Causes stomach issues like reflux, stomach cramps, and nausea.
- Affects the reproductive system by lowering the sperm count of men and reducing sex drive for both men and women.
- Increases your blood pressure and cholesterol, increasing the likelihood of heart attack.
- Creates digestive issues like irritable bowel syndrome (IBS), constipation, and diarrhea.
- Causes unstable moods and behaviors, depression, sleep issues, anxiety disorders, panic attacks, headaches, and low energy.

SELF-LOVE AND CARE

"Love yourself unconditionally, just as you love those closest to you despite their faults."

—LES BROWN

To achieve a mind, body, and soul connection, you must practice self-love and self-care.

My first attempt at practicing self-love was shopping for myself. I soon realized that buying myself material goods I did not need *did not* equal true happiness. Now, when I shop for myself, I call it conscious indulgence. I am no longer oblivious to what I am doing or how it is making me feel. Instead, I make an empowered choice to indulge, rather than a reactive impulse resulting from stress and unhappiness.

When you become conscious about an indulgence, you are less inclined to indulge as often. For example, shopping provided a temporarily fun release for me, but it was not going to change my state of being, nor was it sustainable. Now, when I shop from time to time, I do it consciously. I recognize when an indulgence becomes too much. If I do feel the need to overindulge on a regular basis, I try and identify the underlying cause driving that behavior.

Be careful to distinguish between conscious indulgence and self-medication. Some people use food, drugs, or alcohol to soothe their anxiety or escape reality. People eat without being hungry to fill a void and cope with emotional trauma. You want to replace any of these self-medicating habits with healthy behaviors, like yoga, Pilates, or meditation.

In a way, we are all fighting for life. I am not afraid of dying, and I know there is still so much life out there for me to live. If you constantly look to escape your reality, clearly there is a disconnect between your behavior and your desire to live. Instead of trying to escape your reality, you can find a sustainable way to change it.

SLEEP IS A LONG VERSION OF MEDITATION

"True silence is the rest of the mind, and is to the spirit what sleep is to the body, nourishment and refreshment."

—WILLIAM PENN

Although sleep is such a basic part of life, many of us suffer from insomnia or interrupted sleep. As part of our modern lifestyle, our new norm is to take a sleeping pill like Ambien. Instead of finding the root cause of our insomnia, we are freely prescribed these sleeping pills, and before you know it, we are addicted to taking them every night. By now, I hope you know relying on chemicals to compensate for unhealthy habits is a bad practice.

Cancer patients usually do not sleep well, which is harmful

because sleep allows our bodies to repair and renew damaged cells. When I struggled to sleep, I was thankful for cannabis. Taking it helped me in many ways, so never say never. I remembered lecturing my children to never take cannabis, yet there I was, their own mother, consuming so much of it that I even created my own suppository.

Trying cannabis was an important part of staying openminded about anything that would help me live. When I decided to live, it not only meant creating a limitless attitude, but most importantly, it meant being fearless about trying different things that could potentially help get rid of the tumors in my upper body. Cannabis has medicinal benefits, yet it seems like few people know about this natural therapy available to us, especially people in California, where marijuana is legal.

In my case, I used cannabis as a medicinal treatment because a high dose on a regular basis is known to dissolve tumors. When I heard this, I went full force. In retrospect, I am convinced that using cannabis is how I stayed calm, almost pain free, almost anxiety free, and got plenty of sleep! Is there anything else you know of that gives you all of these benefits without causing real harm to your body? Cannabis is a plant, and taking it was a win-win. It calmed my mind, freed me from any worries associated with the stress of having cancer, and helped me get twelve to fifteen hours of sleep every night. Getting plenty of sleep was extraordinary for my healing.

Why is sleep so important—perhaps even more critical than getting proper nutrition? Sleep affects the body in so many ways, especially glucose and insulin levels. While we sleep, hormones are released, damaged tissues get repaired, detoxification becomes possible, and most importantly, the immune system is restored. If you do not practice good sleep hygiene and deprive yourself of sleep on a regular basis, then it's time you find a solution that works for you as soon as possible. Your mind and body can't benefit from any of your other treatments unless you are able to sleep.

What can you do to make sure you sleep every night? Adopt rituals. Rituals are important as our bodies thrive on routines. My bedroom is a sacred place for me. I make sure everything is conducive to good sleeping hygiene. Absolutely no bright lights after 7:00 p.m., and my phone is not in my bedroom. I use essential oils like lavender or frankincense in a diffuser, and I take a nice warm shower in the dark with calm meditative music before bedtime. I take my supplements (melatonin, cortisol manager, and magnesium) one hour before sleeping.

CREATE A LIFESTYLE OF PURPOSE

"The pain that you've been feeling can't compare to the joy that's coming."

—ROMANS 8:18

In order to live a true, authentic life, you must work towards a **purposeful** life.

I firmly believe in a higher power and spiritual universe, so I never feel alone. I know someone is watching over me and helping to guide me in the right direction. The less present I am, the less I feel God's generous grace. For that reason, I practice meditation to be as mindful and present as possible. Throughout my healing process, I have been guided by overwhelming amounts of grace. God builds our faith by constantly showing us he is with us. When I receive God's grace, the sensation runs through my entire body; sometimes I feel cold, and sometimes I feel like someone has covered me with a heavy blanket.

I cannot take credit for everything that has happened to me. God planned this journey for me because he knew I would be relentless in figuring out a way to be alive and thriving again. God also knew that I would not stop at helping myself get rid of this disease, but that I would have the heart to help others figure it out, too. This process has massively reinforced my faith in God and life itself.

Remember: cancer is not a conspiracy against you—it is a gift. Today, I never worry about what will happen next, because I know I am living a purposeful life and my story has already been written.

DEVELOP YOUR SUPERPOWER: MEDITATION

"Meditation is a vital way to purify and quiet the mind, thus rejuvenating the body."

—DEEPAK CHOPRA

I wake up every day feeling excited about the ability to nourish, challenge, and expand my mind. For me, journaling has become an emotional cleansing. I journal in order to download my emotions and toxic thoughts and to practice gratitude. Writing my top three reasons to be grateful instantly puts a smile on my face. By the end of this ten-minute process, I feel much lighter and calm. **This is when I know I am ready to meditate.**

There are many good reasons to learn to meditate. Every day, we have so many thoughts racing in our minds, and what do you think this does to the body? It creates stress! Meditation is essential because through this practice, you will gain peace of mind, and you will be less anxious and reactive throughout the day. Like any skill, meditation takes practice. Do not judge yourself! When I first started meditating, I often fell asleep. I thought I was not meditating correctly. Quite the contrary! The body is a smart machine, and it was doing what it needed to do at that moment, which was to rest. **Your body is intuitive enough to know what you need at any given moment.**

By the time I finished all my meditation training sessions,

I was not falling asleep anymore. My mind started wandering, and the key when this happens is to be aware of it. This is what it means to be mindful, so celebrate it because most people think this is a sign of a failed meditation session. On the contrary, if you can get to this level of consciousness, then you are doing good. When you notice your mind starting to wander, just bring yourself back to your breath or mantra, which I will discuss later in this chapter. You are exercising being kind to yourself and increasing self-compassion, which is a beautiful thing.

Do not be hard on yourself if you can't do this right away. Meditation takes practice, and most importantly, compassion. Remember, you are committed to doing this for life, so be patient with yourself. One day, you will meditate and realize that you remained present and completely detached yourself from your surroundings, which is very freeing.

By focusing on my breathing and being present, I have become aware of how my body is feeling and have learned to calm my mind to the point where I do not even think of anything. This is when you know you have detached yourself from your thoughts and emotions that create suffering. Your mind feels empty. You experience a sense of relief, peace, and just **good**! Trust me. Not only do you feel the stress leave your body, but the deep breathing gives oxygen to your cells and boosts your immune system. This type of relaxation, which takes no more than ten to fifteen minutes, immensely benefits your body.

BALANCE IS NATURAL

"To a mind that is still, the whole universe surrenders."

—LAO TZU

We all crave happiness. However, we cannot feel happy all the time—nor are we meant to. Accepting the natural balance of emotions can actually help you be more at peace because you will not constantly chase an impossible state of perpetual happiness.

Unhappiness does not equal failure. In fact, you must experience bad times to appreciate the good. When you know how it feels to be in the dark, you celebrate the times when you have light. Nothing is permanent, everything will pass, and even the darkest nights are broken by daylight. Receiving a cancer diagnosis often sends people into a state of depression, but that is not all there is to life. **You are not your diagnosis. This dark time will pass. According to ancient Chinese philosopher Lao Tzu, "New beginnings are often disguised as painful endings."**

God will not give you anything you cannot handle. In my experience, God interrupted the life I had planned for myself. Clearly, he had bigger plans for me. God had faith that I would figure it out, so I started a healing process of self-discovery, which culminated in me writing this book.

Whatever treatment protocol you create, you are going inside your body and mind and getting to the root cause of your problems. You can also treat your hidden wounds with spirituality. As a practice, spirituality teaches you to go deep within yourself and have the difficult conversations you have likely delayed because of fear, laziness, or sleepwalking through life. Spirituality can help you discover *why* you exist, which in turn will shape your lifestyle. If you exist to help others, you must build a lifestyle around that goal—but only after you have helped yourself first. Through augmenting your awareness, self-reflection, taking responsibility for all your actions and words, and honesty, you will learn who you are, what you are made of, and the purpose of you being on this Earth.

Throughout this process, you are not alone: God and the universe will help guide you, but you need to ask the questions and want the answers. When you discover who you are, you give yourself the gift of life—a renewed life where you are fully aware that you are not the same person you were at the time of the cancer diagnosis. The things you argued and fought about are replaced by silence. Now, you are speaking the truth instead of maintaining the status quo. Now, you realize you are unshakeable because you no longer waste your time, energy, and focus on things and people that do not align with your healthy mind and lifestyle. In fact, don't be surprised if you notice a shift in your environment as you shift yourself, because you are not the same person you were before.

The day will come when you wake up and everything feels right, perhaps for the first time in your life. Your heart will be full. Your soul will be smiling. Your thoughts will be positive and strong. Your vision will be crystal clear. You will be calm and at peace with who you have become, where your journey has taken you, and what cancer has put you through. Most importantly, you will be at peace and excited about where you are going.

CANCER IS LIFE CHANGING BUT NOT LIFE DEFINING

"Waking up to who you are requires letting go of who you imagine yourself to be."

—ALAN WATTS

Shortly after my diagnosis and gloomy prognosis, I turned to inspiring books, philosophers, and spiritual teachers for hope. I remember reading one quote from Frederick Lenz, a spiritual Buddhist teacher who said, "Duality is part of reality, and there is definitely winning and losing. If you don't think so, talk to someone who has beaten cancer and talk to somebody who hasn't."

Going from athletic and strong to skin and bones forced me to accept the natural concept of duality that exists in nature and in us.

We see this concept at work in trees every year. Trees can look so beautiful during spring and summer. In winter, most trees go through an ugly period. Some need to be strategically pruned. We are all like trees.

As Lewis Carroll wrote in *Alice's Adventures in Wonderland,* "It's no use going back to yesterday, because I was a different person then."

Right now, I am not the strongest I have ever been. In the past, I have lived a life of physical strength, and now is my time to live a life of acceptance. I have learned to make peace with my past because I know that if I don't, it will ruin my future. I had to work very hard to accept what is today, let go of what was, and have faith and believe in what my future will be. No matter whether I am physically strong or weak, I want to live a life that makes me smile. That joy is part of my daily gift I give to myself, to the people that hover over me, and the people I encounter in my beautiful journey.

I embrace sadness so I can cherish the moments of happiness even more. I live a life of *wabi-sabi* that celebrates the beauty in the imperfections, where I am committed to being courageous, finding the good in the bad, and accepting the cycle of life, which includes death. My goal is to have the life of my dreams by accumulating as many experiences as possible that honor my life's purpose—and by remembering that impossible can be transformed to *I'm possible.*

You can embrace imperfections by honoring your scars. Any soldier who has fought in the military will have badges of honor. If you strip away those badges, the soldier will have scars that tell stories. Clearly, that soldier has lived! They have suffered, been lonely, and been through the unimaginable to discover their greatness. What makes you think you can't be this person? What makes you think that all this pain, brokenness, trauma, and devastation isn't what will fuel and propel you to be your most powerful version of you? **These challenges are your teachers.** Learn their lessons so that they can be your grace.

Dying is as much a part of life as being born. In between those two events, you feel an entire spectrum of emotions every day. Living requires you to reset, adjust, restart, and refocus, not once but many times during your lifetime. Every time you elevate your life, it will demand different things from you. Be ready. Resisting will only delay your growth. Life is not one dimensional, nor does it follow one straight path.

I hope you can make peace with the idea that cancer is not

a death sentence. Trust me, nobody is after you or trying to condemn you. This is not a punishment—see it as part of your story. Have you thought that perhaps God and the universe give the most challenging and, at times, most painful battles to the strongest soldiers? Some leaves fall off tree branches, some turn yellow. Think of this period in your life as an opportunity to figure out *why* you were given cancer. Only you can find the answer to that question.

Cancer is my grace, and it can be yours, too. On the other side of this hurdle stands the person you are supposed to be in this lifetime. You have a responsibility to process the things that happen to you, good and bad, and use them to shape your direction in life. Obviously, you can respond to your cancer diagnosis in a negative way and think of it as a hateful punishment from a vengeful God. However, remember that your interpretations of reality *shape* your reality. Only by keeping a positive mindset and believing in yourself can you heal.

SHAPING YOUR DAILY ROUTINE

You chose to live and to not be discouraged by your Western doctors and the statistics they shared with you. Congratulations in setting the intention to take control of your life instead of allowing somebody else to make the choice for you. It is important to plan the life you want. Be deliberate. An established daily routine is key to healing and should be incorporated in your treatment protocols.

Routines can be powerful as they set your daily habits and reinforce the intention to heal your mind, body, and soul. When you are sick, with so many overwhelming uncertainties, a daily routine helps with anxiety because it puts control back in your court.

Here is an example of my daily routine that you can use for inspiration when designing your own:

- While still in bed, I do a mental and physical scan. I check what I am thinking and if I am experiencing any physical pain.
- I talk to God. I thank God for giving me another day and another chance to show him that I am loving myself and enjoying life to the fullest. I ask God to guide me throughout the day. I thank God that I am able to breathe. I am grateful for whatever God has planned for me for that day.
- I enjoy a huge shot of laughter by listening to a comedy show while I get ready for my day.
- I drink hot water with organic lemon to balance the pH level in my body.
- I drink green juice (without apple because it has an abundance of sugar) to get vitamins and minerals.
- I take time to write in my journal because it de-clutters my mind and removes the negative and recycled thoughts. I reassure myself that no matter how bad my life may seem, I know there is only one thing we are guaranteed: change. I tell myself that

the rainbow will come soon after the rain, and I keep taking steps forward. I journal about my health, and I write that my body is strong and can handle anything. I tell my body to get rid of all the tumors. I write about how I plan to spend my day full of love from family and friends.

- I take a moment to visualize the day and **smile**.
- I eat breakfast, which is usually soup. I alternate between green vegetable soup, carrot ginger soup, and lentil soup.
- I go outside for a walk. Whenever possible, I spend time in nature. I do grounding exercises at the Santa Monica beach where my feet have direct contact with the surface of the earth. Taking these contemplative walks close to nature is known to boost the immune system, help with insomnia, reduce stress, and help with inflammation.
- I feed my brain by studying and reading about the subject of cancer and health.
- I have lunch with loved ones and make sure we are laughing. Laughter, or Vitamin L as I say, is medicine, so make sure you get plenty of it. Surround yourself with people who are a bit crazy and do not take themselves seriously. These are the people you can't replace in life.
- Lunch is usually a raw salad, and I bring my own dressing.
- I usually take naps whenever I am tired.
- Whenever I eliminate waste, I remind myself that cancer cells and toxins are leaving my body.
- I listen to music while I cook dinner. I enter a whole new world with music. Music feeds my heart and soothes my mind. When my mind is overloaded, music empties my head. It is one of the few things that quiets my mind and, at times, makes me forget everything. I close my eyes, blast my music, and enjoy a good date night with myself.
- My dinner is usually a light meal so my body will not be burdened with digesting a lot of food overnight. I believe the less burden my body experiences

during the night, the more it can allocate its energy to healing.

- I follow the sleep hygiene practice of showering before going to bed.
- In bed, before sleeping, I analyze my day. I talk to God and review my day with him. I thank God for giving me the energy I had for that day. I usually tell him, "God, I lived today to the fullest with a purpose, wouldn't you agree? So, don't you think I have earned another day? Please give me another day tomorrow, and I promise to continue to earn my day by being kind to myself and living a healthy lifestyle."
- Lastly, I visualize and talk to the tumors in my body. I remind cancer that I am strong, and I tell it to **get out of my body**!

EXERCISE YOUR BODY

"Be grateful that you can exercise."

—VERONICA VILLANUEVA

Along with mindfulness, good sleep, and other stress-reducing practices like music, time in nature, and art, your new lifestyle should include exercise. Exercise is important for the healing process, especially when you are in remission. Our bodies are meant to move. You only get one body so take great care of it! People tend to take exercise for granted when they can do it without thinking, but when you are sick, even the smallest movements can become hard. I will never again take walking, running, tennis, and all other exercises for granted. The ability to exercise is a gift—if you are able to do so, do not waste yours!

Whether you're fighting an illness or not, everyone can benefit from the health-boosting effects of exercise, including the following:

- Reduces stress
- Causes sweating, which removes toxins from the body
- Expels excess energy from your body, which regulates your sleep cycle and helps with insomnia
- Keeps your insulin levels down
- Gives your immune system a powerful boost
- Stimulates your lymphatic system, which transports infection-fighting white blood cells throughout the body

With so many exercise options to choose from, you want to pick activities you enjoy that feel good for your body's unique needs. For example, I do Pilates because the movements quiet my mind and allow me to focus only on my breathing and form. The stretching involved in Pilates reduces my stress, improves my circulation, and releases my stiffness. I do not do yoga because many of the positions that require bending over hurt due to the two scars below my right breast where I had surgery to drain the cancer fluid from my lungs. This is what works for my body, but you might find that yoga or other exercises work best for you.

Do what you can, even if that means only going for a

short twenty- or thirty-minute walk. Walking for me was a lesson in humility. I went from playing competitive tennis and being able to deadlift 125 pounds to barely being able to breathe. I will never take my physical strength for granted again.

To have a healthy lifestyle that is sustainable, you must invest in yourself. Being well is an **active** process. Remember, like any other goal, you need to really want it in order to be successful. Wellness is not confined to a single area; a healthy lifestyle is medicine.

Some of the tools discussed in this book might not be relevant for you today. My advice is to not discard them. Chances are that at some point in the future one or more of these tools *will* become relevant in your life. Think of these recommendations as a comfort for moments of uncertainty. My aim is to provide reassurance and reinforce the fact that **I am alive** today, despite the odds I was given. There is always a way, and it is your responsibility to find your way to healing. Sometimes when I see a weed growing in between cracks in cement, I identify with it because that was me. Like a weed—tough, persistent, and adaptable—I have learned to grow in any environment after a cancer diagnosis. Join me in proving that we, too, against all odds, can bloom into a beautiful flower!

As Helen Keller said, "A happy life consists not in the absence, but in the mastery of hardships."

Your new life can only be exposed by giving up the old one. We cannot become what we are meant to be if we do not detach from who we were. Maybe cancer was not meant to disrupt your life but to clear your path. Where will you go next?

FIND YOUR MANTRA

"The main purpose of life is to live rightly, think rightly, act rightly. The soul must languish when we give all our thought to the body."

—MAHATMA GANDHI

Every time I walk into an oncologist appointment, I repeat my mantra: *respirez...tout ira bien...BELIEVE.* This means, *breathe...everything will be fine...BELIEVE,* in French.

What prompted me to create a mantra?

As I described earlier in the book, when I first began getting CT scans of my chest, pelvis, and abdomen every quarter, I felt so scared and impatient to know my results. I didn't realize my oncologist was not in the office on Fridays, which meant I had to wait until after the weekend to hear my results. This waiting was complete torture for me. I remember feeling frustrated and overwhelmed with anxiety. Three days seemed so far away.

It was at this moment I realized I had disempowered and allowed myself to feel the "unnecessary" anxiety plaguing my mind and body. I thought, *this can't be good for me*. I was continuing to make myself sick by having these self-induced negative emotions. I also realized I would be getting CT scans frequently, and I couldn't imagine going through that each time. I decided my mindset had to evolve. I needed something to calm me down.

So, I changed the way I saw the situation. I thought, *there is nothing I can do about the results. It's done. The results are recorded, and my worrying and frustration will not change what the doctor will tell me when he interprets the findings.*

I needed to learn to surrender and **believe** that no matter what the results were, I was going to **live**!

The results meant nothing because I would continue to do everything I could to get rid of the tumors that covered my upper body. If I truly believed that I was here to stay, the scan results should not matter. From that day forward, I decided to always make my scan appointments on Thursdays so I'd be forced to wait patiently for a few days and be at peace while waiting. This was the first time in my life I had made the conscious decision to embrace being uncomfortable and to actually go after something I was not good at and feared. I journaled a list of all the things

I needed to be better at, and next to it, I wrote a plan to replace those negative behaviors with positive ones.

Next, I created my mantra to support my vision—to live—and to help me find peace. Every time I entered my oncologist's office, I would take a deep breath and repeat my mantra. In the beginning, my breathing was so shallow due to my right lung's inability to work as well as it did before the diagnosis. I reminded myself that because God and the universe love me, everything would be fine. I had to BELIEVE not only in everything great I had been doing to heal myself, but also in the higher power "hovering over me," as author Carolyn Myss says, ready to protect me. In April 2019, my first scan of the year, I decided to have my next scan not in four months, but in eight months! To me, this is what it meant to believe in myself and in the higher power.

Since creating my mantra, which is stenciled on my wall in front of my desk, I have repeated those words, *respirez... tout ira bien...BELIEVE (breathe...everything will be fine... BELIEVE)*, every time I start to feel fear and anxiety. It is amazing how this mantra has helped me be in the present and replaced the negative thoughts with positivity.

JOURNAL EXERCISE: CRAFT YOUR MANTRA

Whenever I go to get scan results, my mantra helps me imagine myself as "Veronica's best friend," not Veronica herself. I separate myself from the mindset of the patient so I can stay calm and pragmatic, ask all the right questions, and keep emotion out of the equation. Ironically, a breath is always the starting point for almost anything I do, yet I struggled with not being able to breathe correctly in the early days after the diagnosis.

I suggest that you create a mantra because, at times, you will feel anxious and overwhelmed during your healing journey. You need to get comfortable with "the unknown." Your mantra will stop all the brain chatter that only produces negative emotions. Your mantra will keep you from worrying about the future.

Let's face it, every time we think about the future, we worry. The minute you start to feel out of control and overwhelmed, activate your mantra. It is like magic. It brings you to the present moment, which is where you need to be. Focus replaces anxiety.

When you are learning to be mindful, you need a mantra that means something significant to *you*. Brainstorm in your journal and write down options until a certain word or phrase speaks to you and makes you feel empowered.

Your mantra is very personal. The goal is to make you feel more secure during a moment of uncertainty. I suggest you think of a short sentence that is powerful enough to awaken you to the present moment when anxiety and fear want to take over. Think of something that will empower and comfort you instantly once you whisper your mantra to yourself. Remember, when you repeat your mantra to yourself, you are practicing replacing negativity with positivity.

_____

ON TOP OF THE MOUNTAIN

"The greatest gift you have to give is that of your own transformation."

—LAO TZU

A transformed and enlightened person has the power to create a better world. When you experience spiritual evolution, you learn to empower yourself and improve your ability to navigate through the hurdles of life while remaining unshakeable. When you understand who you are, that you are meant to shift to a higher level, your energy in the universe and around you will drastically change. Dale Carnegie once said, "Most of the important things in the world have been accomplished by people who kept on trying when there seemed to be no hope at all." So, *be* the change the world needs.

Today, as I stand on top of my mountain having reached my goal, **to live**, I see life as a gift. A new life, a new way of living is meaningless without many moments of *metanoia*, which means a spiritual conversion or journey of changing one's mind, heart, self, or way of life. As my level of consciousness has heightened, I have gained an understanding of the difference between *a* reality and *the* reality. I feel privileged that I am able to redesign my life with an enlightened mind. After reading this book, my hope is that you too feel enlightened and inspired to experience a similar transformation.

Nobody expects to be diagnosed with cancer. However, once you accept your diagnosis and learn to be at peace with it, you can empower yourself toward healing. This positive change ignites a ripple effect, and you can use your enlightenment to help other people, which is what I hope to have done by writing this book.

The overflowing grace I have witnessed in my experience is an opportunity to help you strengthen your muscle of hope. Cancer is **not** a death sentence. View this as your metanoia, your journey to change your mind, heart, self, and way of life. Challenges, from getting divorced to being diagnosed with cancer, present opportunities for healing and expansion, but too often, people do not connect the dots. Embrace this experience and believe that something beautiful is about to happen. Remember, we do not grow when things come easy; we grow when we face challenges and push through pain. This is your chance to go on a journey of self-discovery that will pave your path to transformation. You, too, are about to witness the grace of cancer.

TODAY, IS CANCER CURABLE?

"You gain strength, courage, and confidence by every experience in which you really stop to look fear in the face. You are able to say to yourself, I lived through this horror. I can take the next thing that comes along. You must do the thing you think you cannot do."

—ELEANOR ROOSEVELT

Although my treatment and experience are unique to me, there are certain lifestyle factors, like chronic stress and a poor diet, that many of us have in common. By reading this book, you have acquired the tools to replace habits that no longer serve you, **and you have taken control of your life.** You have taken proactive steps toward healing. You have refused to be a victim of a disease by taking actions. The voice inside your head that told you to pick up this book is the grace of cancer.

In your moments of doubt, remind yourself what it means to **be alive.** Ask yourself, is each day fuller than it was yesterday? If you only have six months to live, what kind of life do you want to have? When you allow cancer to control your mind, body, and soul, you become a victim of the disease. Instead of playing the victim, educate yourself about the process of healing. You are given this life because you are courageous enough to live it! Get excited about redesigning your life because the only way it gets better is by changing.

If your environment got you sick in the first place, it is the first thing that needs to change. In the words of Einstein, "The definition of insanity is doing the same thing over and over again and expecting a different result." Stop making the same old mistakes that made you sick.

In your life, it is not the external events themselves that cause distress. It is the way you think about these events. Train your mind to see the positive in every situation. It all comes down to your interpretation and response to the events in your life. Your happiness depends on the quality of your thoughts. We cannot choose our external circumstances; challenges and unpleasant situations are inevitable in life. For example, you cannot control your cancer diagnosis. However, you *can* control how you respond to that diagnosis. Once you accept your circumstances, you can change the way you think about them. **Maybe, just maybe, this disease is trying to teach you something.**

When I say cancer is treatable, not everybody believes me. But I only speak from experience. The more I study cancer, the more I have learned about the amazing progress that has been made. In most cases, a percentage of treatments fail to work, but I believe part of that comes down to human resistance and not being mentally and emotionally open to trying everything. Throughout this healing process, you need to open yourself up to **all** the possibilities to help yourself.

THE PRICE OF TRANSFORMATION

"If you really want to escape the things that harass you, what you're needing is not to be in a different place but to be a different person."

—SENECA

Transformation cannot take place without pain and struggle. This journey will be difficult at times, but it is temporary. The pain, challenges, and struggles will all be worth it for the incredible life you are building for yourself. **Believe** in the opportunity to grow and become a better version of yourself.

Right now, you are living. You are not sleepwalking through your own life, like so many others are doing, fearful of any experiences that come their way. A full life is limitless, and that includes a wide spectrum of experiences and emotions, including pain. However, to live a full life, you cannot be paralyzed by your emotions. It is not wrong to feel fear, but you must turn that fear into drive and determination to achieve your goals.

Healing is hard work, but I will always be grateful for the chance to better myself and my life. Imagine how good it feels to overcome all the things that were supposed to destroy you!

FIND HOPE

"However bad life may seem, there is always something you can do and succeed at. Where there's life, there's hope."

—STEPHEN HAWKING

Now, it is your turn to develop your muscle of hope. That hope will fuel your healing, growth, and transformation, especially when the future feels darkest.

When I tell my story, people often ask me what I did to be alive today. My answer? The solution is never just one thing. I transformed my entire lifestyle, and I cannot say for certain which changes helped more than others, only that the cumulative effect of all my efforts healed me.

I am positive the reason I am still here today is because I did not think about dying. My belief in myself and my life has always been stronger than any negative thoughts. I only surrounded myself with people who believed in me enough to take part in and support my healing journey.

Today, all that matters is that I feel good, happy, and healthy. Right now, I am doing exactly what I want in life. It does not matter that I am not officially "in remission." It matters that I am living and breathing when all the doctors said I was not supposed to be.

Nobody knows how much time they have on this earth. Cancer did *not* come into my life to scare me into thinking I would die tomorrow. The universe gave me cancer to teach me about my potential, humility, and greatness, and to live the best life possible.

Now that I have experienced cancer, I do not pretend it never happened. I live as mindfully as I can to keep the disease from returning. With the knowledge, recognition, and respect I now have for my body, I am motivated to live a healthier and more sustainable lifestyle.

My hope is that you can learn from my experience without having to go through the disease yourself.

YOUR STORY, YOUR TURN

Reading this book is not enough to change you. This book will only change you if you actively **want** to change. Everyone has their own timeline, and this was mine.

In the beginning of this book, I asked you to create a vision of yourself making the decision to live. Now, return to that vision. Imagine you are already at the top of your mountain. Believe, pray, and manifest every goal in your beautiful life.

The journey will be difficult, but it will be worth every second. You need to balance your body and boost your immune system to prevent cancer from thriving inside you. However, your mind is equally as important to healing as your body. **Focus on mastering an open and expansive mind.**

Together, let's change the statistics around cancer. I want *you* to help me prove cancer doesn't have to be a death sentence. Let's start a trend where doctors share positive statistics and list natural and effective therapies as a key component to any healing protocol. Let's plant the seed of hope for people who are devastated by their cancer diagnosis. Once you are standing on top of your mountain, I want to hear your story, too.

LOOKING TOWARD THE FUTURE

"A hero is no braver than an ordinary man, but he is brave five minutes longer."

—RALPH WALDO EMERSON

As the designers at Bryan Anthonys wrote for their Drop of Hope design, "Ditch logic. Ditch the odds. Hold on to hope, even if this is just a single drop. The universe loves a persistent heart. I do not know what will happen to me, but the words 'I give up' will never be part of my language vocabulary."

Whether you follow some or all of my advice, I hope that this book has helped you realize **you can fight this disease**. Once you make the decision to live, all of the tools are at your disposal. The more you educate yourself, the more you and your team can create aggressive, personalized protocols that work for you. After you start, I encourage you to keep adding to your approach and continuously evolve your cancer-beating strategy.

Rather than stressing, allow the possibility of a transformed life to excite you. When you begin your healing journey according to the recommendations in this book, your energy will surge, and as soon as you assemble the pieces, you will witness magic and miracles.

Now is the time to fill your mind with a real passion for a phenomenal life. If you do not already, try praying or meditating. Make time for love, joy, empowering thoughts, gratitude, family, friends, music, and laughter.

Picture the day of your last scan showing no evidence of disease and **hold on to that image**. That image will be your future if you take responsibility for the life you are creating, use this experience to discover your true purpose, and follow your path to happiness. Once you know your purpose, you will treasure your life more than ever before.

I am stronger because I decided to be.

I am braver because I fought hard and earned my new life.

I am happier because I know what is truly important in life.

I am a badass because I have scars to remind me that I turned pain into my superpower!

It's time to live your best life. Join me!

Appendix A

BOOK RECOMMENDATIONS

"There is no greater agony than bearing an untold story inside you."

—MAYA ANGELOU

Our lives are like books. There are chapters that are happy and some that are sad. It's by turning the pages that we come to a realization that nothing stays constant. Even in books, change is inevitable.

The Grace of Cancer, Veronica Villanueva

Alkaline Herbal Medicine, Aqiyl Aniys

Gerson Therapy, Charlotte Gerson and Morton Walker, D.P.M.

How Not to Die, Michael Greger, MD, Gene Stone

Keto for Cancer, Miriam Kalamian, EdM, MS, CNS, foreword by Thomas N. Seyfried, PhD

The Plant Paradox, Steven R. Gundry, MD

Fat for Fuel, Dr. Joseph Mercola

The Metabolic Approach to Cancer, Dr. Nasa Winters, ND, L.Ac., FABNO, Jess Higgins Kelley, MNT

Sleep Smarter, Shawn Stevenson

The Book of Joy, Dalai Lama, Desmond Tutu, Douglas Abrams

The Book of Awakening, Mark Nepo

The Heart of the Buddha's Teaching, Thich Nhat Hanh

The Art of Power, Thich Nhat Hanh

The Tao of Pooh, Benjamin Hoff

Beyond Fear, Don Miguel Ruiz

The Alchemist, Paulo Coelho

Wabi-Sabi, Leonard Koren

How Your Mind Can Heal Your Body, David R. Hamilton, PhD

A Whole New Mind, Daniel H. Pink

Aware, Daniel J. Siegel, MD

What Makes Us Healthy, Caroline Myss

Exploring Chakras, Caroline Myss

Channeling Grace, Caroline Myss

Happiness, Matthieu Ricard

You Are the Placebo, Joe Dispenza

Seat of the Soul, Gary Zukav

A New Earth, Eckhard Tolle

The Power of Moments, Chip Heath and Dan Heath

The Rumi Daybook, Kabir and Camille Helminski

The Power of Transcendental Meditation, Bob Roth

The Mindful Athlete, George Mumford

How to Change Your Mind, Michael Pollan

Willpower Doesn't Work, Benjamin Hardy

Living in Your Top 1%, Alissa Finerman

Life is What You Make It, Peter Buffett

Appendix B

HEALTHY RECIPES

Try cooking these healthy recipes, each of which is packed full of nutrient-rich foods that will help your body fight disease.

I had very little variety in my diet during the first year and a half after my diagnosis. Most days, I ate the same soup and salad because I believed the constant introduction of new food would require my body to work harder to digest. By keeping my meals simple, nutritious, and familiar, my body could direct more energy toward healing instead of digesting.

CARROT-GINGER SOUP

There are so many health benefits to eating soup, which is why I often eat soup for breakfast, lunch, and dinner. Cooking soup is easy and can keep fresh for days in your refrigerator. The soups I make have a creamy and velvety texture without any dairy by using more vegetables and less broth.

With any recipe, I always make sure to gently cook the vegetables to retain their nutrients. Most cancer patients need to gain healthy weight by consuming food with high amounts of healthy fat and a lot of vegetables (approximately five cups), and soup can help you meet this requirement. Additionally, soup gives you the nutrients you need to fight cancer, raise your strength and energy levels, deal with chemotherapy and radiation side effects, heal and recover faster, and feel better overall.

HEALTH BENEFITS OF EACH INGREDIENT

- Olive oil is a good source of fat.
- Onion helps eliminate toxins and carcinogens. Onion has anti-cancer benefits due to the sulfur compounds known as allicin. The flavonoid quercetin also helps boost your immune system.
- Garlic also has anti-inflammatory benefits. The best part about garlic is that it helps your body kill cancer cells while also boosting the immune system. Avoid overcooking garlic because high temperatures will kill the allicin. For this reason, I always add garlic toward the end of cooking.
- Carrots, despite their sweetness, are packed with disease-fighting nutrients. Beta carotene can help

prevent many diseases and slows down the growth of cancer cells.

- Ginger contains many medicinal properties and has anti-inflammatory benefits. If you are doing chemotherapy, this is a good soup to counter your nausea.
- Apple cider vinegar is known to reduce the insulin levels in people with type 2 diabetes. Additionally, drinking a small amount of apple cider vinegar before a meal decreases your appetite, thereby aiding in weight loss.

CARROT-GINGER SOUP RECIPE

(Serves 3–5)

Ingredients (all organic):

- 1 tablespoon extra virgin olive oil
- 2 red onions, chopped
- 5 stalks of celery, chopped
- 7 garlic cloves, minced
- 4 cups carrots, chopped (medium size cubes)
- 1 ¾ teaspoons grated fresh ginger
- 1 tablespoon apple cider vinegar
- 4 cups vegetable broth (less if thicker soup is desired)
- ½ teaspoon of Himalayan pink salt
- 1 teaspoon of black pepper

Preparation:

- Heat the olive oil in a large soup pot over medium heat. Add the onions, salt, and pepper and cook until softened, stirring occasionally, about 7 minutes. Add the carrots to the pot and cook about 10 minutes, stirring occasionally.
- Add the ginger, garlic, apple cider vinegar, and then 4 cups of broth, depending on your desired consistency. Simmer and cook until the carrots are soft, about 20 minutes.
- Let cool and transfer to a blender. Blend until smooth. Do not add all the broth if you want the soup to be thick. Taste and adjust seasonings.
- Add crushed walnuts on top and garnish with parsley. (Optional)

BROCCOLI-AND-SPINACH SOUP

Eating this soup is a great way to add more green vegetables to your diet.

HEALTH BENEFITS OF EACH INGREDIENT

- Coconut oil is a good source of dietary fat that helps your body burn fat and nourishes the brain.
- Onion helps eliminate toxins and carcinogens. Onion has anti-cancer benefits due to the sulfur compounds

known as allicin. The flavonoid quercetin also helps boost your immune system.

- Garlic also has anti-inflammatory benefits. The best part about garlic is that it helps your body kill cancer cells while also boosting the immune system. Avoid overcooking garlic because high temperatures will kill the allicin. For this reason, I always add garlic toward the end of cooking.
- Broccoli is a cruciferous vegetable that has anti-inflammatory benefits and contains cancer-fighting properties. It is known to boost the body's enzymes and clean out the cancer-causing chemicals in the body.
- Apple cider vinegar is known to reduce the insulin levels in people with type 2 diabetes. Additionally, drinking a small amount of apple cider vinegar before a meal decreases your appetite, thereby aiding in weight loss.
- Coconut milk has MCT oil, which is a good source of fat that promotes weight loss.
- Spinach is a dark, leafy vegetable that protects the body from free radicals.
- Parsley is my herb of choice because it has so many health benefits. Known to help with skin cancer, parsley also strengthens the immune system, is good for the bones, and was used in place of antibiotics.

BROCCOLI-AND-SPINACH SOUP RECIPE

(Serves 3–5)

Ingredients (all organic):

- 1 tablespoon coconut oil, plus extra for garnish
- 2 red onions, chopped
- 2 stems of leeks, chopped
- 5 stalks of celery, diced
- 7 garlic cloves, minced
- 2 heads of broccoli
- 1 ½ teaspoons apple cider vinegar
- 3 cups of vegetable broth (4 cups if not using coconut milk)
- 1 cup light coconut milk (optional)
- 4 cups of spinach
- ½ teaspoon of Himalayan pink salt
- 1 teaspoon of black pepper
- Fresh parsley

Preparation:

- Cut off the green part of the leeks. Slice the white and light green parts vertically in half then turn over for stability before cutting into half rings. Soak in water to remove all the sand. Wash and strain at least twice. Dry thoroughly before cooking.
- Heat the coconut oil in a large pot over medium heat.

Add the onions, leeks, salt, and pepper. Stir until both the onions and leeks are soft, about 7 minutes.

- Chop the broccoli, including the stems, add to the pot. Stir and cook until just softened, about 2 minutes.
- Add the garlic, apple cider vinegar, and then 3 cups of vegetable broth, depending on your desired consistency. Simmer and cook for 4 minutes.
- Add 1 cup of coconut milk if desired. Simmer for 2 minutes.
- Allow the soup to cool down.
- Work in batches. Combine the spinach and soup in a blender. Blend until desired texture. The smoother, the better.
- Garnish with a drizzle of coconut milk and olive oil. Sprinkle with red pepper flakes, if desired. Optionally garnish with a little more coconut milk and add crushed walnuts and fresh parsley.

LENTIL SOUP

This recipe will help you eat more legumes, which can aid in muscle-mass growth.

HEALTH BENEFITS OF EACH INGREDIENT

- Olive oil is a good source of fat.
- Onion helps eliminate toxins and carcinogens. Onion has anti-cancer benefits due to the sulfur compounds

known as allicin. The flavonoid quercetin also helps boost your immune system.

- Celery is a miracle food. I add celery in every dish I prepare, whether cooked or raw salads. It contains an anti-cancer compound called apigenin, which causes the cancer cells to self-destruct (apoptosis).
- Garlic also has anti-inflammatory benefits. The best part about garlic is that it helps your body kill cancer cells while also boosting the immune system. Avoid overcooking garlic because high temperatures will kill the allicin. For this reason, I always add garlic toward the end of cooking.
- Broccoli is a cruciferous vegetable that has anti-inflammatory benefits and contains cancer-fighting properties. It is known to boost the body's enzymes and clean out the cancer-causing chemicals in the body.
- Apple cider vinegar is known to reduce the insulin levels in people with type 2 diabetes. Additionally, drinking a small amount of apple cider vinegar before a meal decreases your appetite, thereby aiding in weight loss.
- Coconut milk has MCT oil, which is a good source of fat that promotes weight loss.
- Lentils are legumes. All legumes should be soaked for at least twenty-four hours in the refrigerator to help address the issue of lectin. Lentils are a great source of fiber as well as plant-based proteins. While I did not eat any animal protein, I ate a lot of legumes to gain muscle mass.

- Spinach is a dark, leafy vegetable that protects the body from free radicals.
- Parsley is my herb of choice because it has so many health benefits. Known to help with skin cancer, parsley also strengthens the immune system, is good for the bones, and was used in place of antibiotics.

LENTIL SOUP RECIPE

(Serves 3–5)

Ingredients (all organic):

- 2 tablespoons extra-virgin olive oil
- 2 cups chopped onions
- 4 stalks of celery, plus chopped celery leaves for garnish
- 1 ½ cup carrots, chopped
- 5 garlic cloves, minced
- 1 tablespoon of apple cider vinegar (optional)
- 4 cups vegetable broth, (more if needed)
- 1 ¾ cups lentils, soaked in water for 24 hours, rinsed, drained
- ½ teaspoon of Himalayan pink salt
- 1 teaspoon of black pepper
- Fresh parsley
- Spinach, add the desired amount at the end, allowing the steam to cook it.

Preparation:

- Heat oil in heavy large saucepan over medium-high heat.
- Add onions until translucent, about 5 minutes.
- Add celery, and carrots. Sauté until vegetables are soft, about 10 minutes.
- Add the lentils, cook for 4 minutes.
- Add ½ teaspoon of Himalayan pink salt.
- Add 1 teaspoon of black pepper.
- Add the apple cider vinegar and broth.
- Reduce heat to medium-low, cover, and simmer until lentils are tender, about 30 minutes. Cook another 5 minutes if you do not like it slightly crunchy.
- Transfer 1 cup of soup (mostly solids) to blender and purée until smooth.
- Return puréed soup in the pot of soup. This should thicken the soup. If too thick, add more broth.
- Remove pot from heat. Add only the desired amount of spinach that you will eat. By allowing the steam to cook the spinach, it helps preserve the nutrients of the vegetable.
- Garnish with fresh chopped parsley.

HARISSA HUMMUS

This recipe makes hummus with a twist of harissa. Harissa is a spicy chili paste extremely popular in North African and

Middle Eastern cuisine. It has a robust and complex flavor. All the spices used in making harissa are antioxidants. A bit of spicy food is good for us because it stimulates our metabolism. You can find harissa in most grocery stores like Whole Foods.

HEALTH BENEFITS OF EACH INGREDIENT

- Chickpeas are part of the legume family. They are a great source of fiber as well as plant-based proteins. While I did not eat any animal protein, I ate a lot of legumes to gain muscle mass. Most importantly, chickpeas have genistein, which is used to treat cancer.
- Harissa is a North African spice. It is also used widely in Middle Eastern dishes, especially in Moroccan food. Harissa is a blend of different spices: dried red chili, garlic paste, caraway, and coriander seed. The spicy chili peppers contain capsaicin, which is anti-inflammatory and antioxidant.
- Cumin is a spice that comes from the Cuminum. It is part of the parsley family. You can find it as whole dried seeds or as ground powder. It aids with digestion and has anti-inflammatory benefits.
- Paprika has carotenoids and beta carotene. These compounds are known to help with oxidative stress, which we now know contributes to cancer.
- Parsley is my herb of choice because it has so many health benefits. Known to help with skin cancer, parsley

also strengthens the immune system, is good for the bones, and was used in place of antibiotics.

Ingredients (all organic):

- 2 cups drained canned chickpeas, liquid set aside
- ¼ cup extra virgin olive oil (optional—Cannabis Infused Oil)
- ½ cup tahini (sesame paste), optional, with some of its oil
- 6 cloves garlic, peeled, depending on how garlicky you want
- 1 teaspoon of harissa (reduce to half for less spice)
- 1 tablespoon of ground cumin
- ½ teaspoon of ground paprika
- Pink Himalayan salt and freshly ground black pepper to taste
- Juice of 1 lemon
- Garnish with fresh chopped parsley

Preparation:

- Combine everything except for the parsley in a food processor. Add the chickpea liquid. Add some alkaline water as needed to get a smooth and consistent purée.
- Taste to see if seasoning needs to be adjusted. Adding more lemon juice at the end is sometimes necessary for a bit of a kick.

- Before serving, drizzle with olive oil and sprinkle with paprika and some parsley.
- Serve with vegetable crudités or cauliflower pizza dough.

CRUNCHY CABBAGE SALAD WITH PROBIOTIC MISO TAHINI DRESSING

Eating this tasty and crunchy salad is a good way to eat more raw vegetables.

HEALTH BENEFITS OF EACH INGREDIENT

- Cabbage has similar health benefits to broccoli since it is from the same plant family, cruciferous. High in beta carotene, fiber, and vitamin C, cabbage also contains sinigrin, which is a must in an anti-cancer diet. Cabbage is another anti-inflammatory and antioxidant ingredient that should be part of any healthy diet. You can eat it raw or cooked.
- Onion helps eliminate toxins and carcinogens. Onion has anti-cancer benefits due to the sulfur compounds known as allicin. The flavonoid quercetin also helps boost your immune system.
- Fennel contains selenium (a mineral in Brazilian nuts) that helps with detoxification, prevents inflammation, and reduces tumor growth.
- Fresh mint is one of my favorite herbs. A fresh mint

tea is my go-to drink at the bar! I get strange looks, but since I do not drink alcohol, I always ask for mint tea in lieu of a cocktail. Mint leaves are known to starve cancer cells by attacking their blood supply! Add as many mint leaves to your salads as you can and drink mint tea all day long.

- Miso, because it is fermented, is packed with "good" bacteria for our gut. No wonder many people in Japan drink miso soup even for breakfast!
- Tahini is a good source of healthy fat with anti-inflammatory, antioxidant properties. It is a great source of calcium. We all suffer from inflammation and should include tahini in our daily diets whenever possible.
- Harissa is a North African spice. It is also used widely in Middle Eastern dishes, especially in Moroccan food. Harissa is a blend of different spices: dried red chili, garlic paste, caraway, and coriander seed. The spicy chili peppers contain capsaicin, which is anti-inflammatory and an antioxidant.
- Cilantro helps get rid of heavy metals in the body. It is full of vitamins and minerals, and is a great source of antioxidants.

Ingredients (all organic):

- ½ green savoy cabbage
- ½ red cabbage

- 1 red onion
- fennel bulb
- 1 cup of fresh mint leaves
- For the miso-tahini dressing:
  - 4 tablespoons white miso
  - 4 tablespoons tahini (choose hulled for a creamier taste)
  - 1 tablespoon freshly grated ginger (I say, the more the merrier)
  - 1 tablespoon Manuka honey
  - 2 tablespoons sesame oil
  - ½ teaspoon of harissa
  - 1 teaspoon of cilantro (Optional)
  - Juice of one lemon

Preparation:

- Shred the onion, cabbage, and fennel. Transfer into a stainless-steel bowl.
- Combine all remaining ingredients to make the dressing. Blend the dressing until smooth.
- Pour desired amount of dressing onto the cabbage.
- Add the fresh mint last so it doesn't bruise when you mix. The best way to mix a salad is by hand. You can use gloves.
- Refrigerate unused dressing.

LEMON VINAIGRETTE DRESSING

I eat a lot of salad, so a healthy salad dressing plays a very important role in my meals! The most important ingredient in a salad dressing is your choice of oil. Some of the olive oils I use are probably more expensive than a bottle of wine. I can justify buying expensive olive oil because I do not drink alcohol. Think of it as oil in your brain. Nothing is too expensive for your brain!

What makes a delicious salad?

Salad starts with the best quality and freshest ingredients. Refer to the list of High-Quality Foods in **Appendix C** for ideas on selecting the different ingredients for your salad. Remember, the more your salad looks like a rainbow, the more balanced it is. Colors, colors, colors make a happy salad!

Texture combined with different flavors should be part of creating a beautiful salad. A good crunch is always a nice surprise when biting into a salad. Another element of surprise could be something spicy at the end of each bite. Paprika and cumin are great spices to incorporate in your dressings.

Don't forget your nuts and seeds: walnuts, pumpkin seeds, pomegranate seeds, and sunflower seeds!

I make all my dressings from scratch and store them in glass canning jars, which I can shake and pour.

Ingredients (all organic):

- 1 cup apple cider vinegar
- 6 tablespoons Dijon mustard
- 2 cups extra virgin olive oil or avocado oil
- Zest and juice of 1 lemon (about 4 tablespoons juice and 3 teaspoons zest)
- 4 clove garlic, finely minced
- 3 tablespoons honey (optional)
- 1 tablespoon of parsley
- 2 teaspoon salt
- 1 teaspoon black pepper
- 3 tablespoon fresh minced oregano

Preparation:

- Combine all ingredients in a jar with a tight-fitting lid and shake. That's it!
- Let it sit for an hour before putting in the refrigerator. This is good for one week. I usually use all of it before the week is up.

V'S GARLIC DRESSING

If you love garlic, this recipe is for you.

Ingredients (all organic):

- 1 cup roasted garlic
- 2 cup avocado oil
- 1 cup apple cider vinegar
- ½ cup of vegetable or bone broth
- ½ teaspoon of paprika
- 1 tablespoon of oregano
- ½ teaspoon of salt
- 1 teaspoon of black pepper

Preparation:

- Combine all the ingredients in a blender or food processor and pulse until smooth.
- Let it sit for an hour before putting in the refrigerator. This is good for one week. I usually use all of it before the week is up.

CANNABIS-INFUSED ORGANIC OLIVE OIL

By infusing cannabis into olive oil, you can easily add cannabis to almost any meal you cook. This recipe takes half an hour to make and lasts for a whole year. One cup of oil will contain approximately 275 milligrams of THC, the compound that causes a "high" and helps fight cancer cells.

The most important ingredient in this recipe is high-quality "cured" cannabis flower. Cured simply means that the internal and external parts of the flower are absolutely dried to prevent breeding mold and fungus, which are toxic.

Ingredients (all organic):

- 1 cup of cured cannabis flowers, finely grounded
- 1 cup of organic extra virgin olive oil
- 1 teaspoon of oregano
- 1 tablespoon of garlic powder
- ½ teaspoon of salt
- 1 teaspoon of pepper
- Cheesecloth
- Finest mesh strainer

Preparation:

- I have a designated cannabis grinder (same as a coffee grinder). Grind the cannabis flower as fine as possible. This is going to be very sticky, so use a silicon spatula to scrape it out completely.
- In a small saucepan, simmer 1 cup of extra virgin olive oil on the lowest heat setting while stirring in the cannabis flower, garlic powder, oregano, salt, and pepper. This should take no more than 15 minutes. Remove from the stove and allow to cool.
- Use either a mason jar or a measuring cup, put a metal strainer on top, and drape a fine mesh over the strainer.

Pour the cannabis-infused olive oil into the mesh and squeeze until there is no more oil coming out of the cheesecloth. Discard the cannabis flower.

- Transfer the cannabis-infused oil to a dark glass bottle using a funnel. Store in a dark and cool place.
- Ideas for usage: any warm or cold salads, pasta sauces, steamed or sautéed vegetables, or protein marinades.

Appendix C

HIGH-QUALITY FOODS

The following lists include nutrient-rich, healthy foods you should work into your diet, from produce, grains, and legumes[16] to proteins, nuts, and fats.[17] Whenever possible, buy organic.

NUTRIENT-RICH FOODS

- Arugula
- Bamboo shoots
- Celery
- Leafy vegetables
- Spinach
- Fresh Parsley
- Fresh Cilantro

16 Li, William W. *Eat to Beat Disease: the New Science of How the Body Can Heal Itself.* New York: Grand Central Publishing, 2019.

17 Kalamian, Miriam. *Keto for Cancer: Ketogenic Metabolic Therapy as a Targeted Nutritional Strategy.* White River Junction, VT: Chelsea Green Publishing, 2017.

- Fresh Mint
- Radishes and daikon
- Summer squash and zucchini
- Carrot
- Fennel
- Garlic
- Green beans
- Mushrooms
- Onion

CANCER-FIGHTING FOODS

- Asparagus
- Belgian endive
- Bok choy
- Broccoli
- Broccoli rabe
- Broccoli sprouts
- Cabbage
- Capers
- Cauliflower
- Celery
- Cherry tomatoes
- Chicory
- Chili peppers
- Collard greens
- Eggplant
- Escarole

- Frisée
- Kale
- Kimchi
- Mustard greens
- Purple potatoes
- Radicchio
- Red-leaf lettuce
- Rutabaga
- San Marzano tomatoes
- Sauerkraut
- Spinach
- Squash blossoms
- Swiss chard
- Tangerine tomatoes
- Turnips
- Wasabi
- Watercress

LEGUMES AND FUNGI

- Black beans
- Chanterelle mushrooms
- Cordyceps
- Chickpeas
- Enoki mushrooms
- Lentils
- Lion's mane
- Maitake

- Morel
- Navy beans
- Oyster mushrooms
- Peas
- Porcini mushrooms
- Shiitake mushrooms
- Soy
- Truffles
- While button mushrooms

SPICES AND HERBS

- Basil
- Cinnamon
- Ginseng
- Licorice root
- Marjoram
- Oregano
- Parsley
- Peppermint
- Rosemary
- Saffron
- Sage
- Thyme
- Turmeric

PROTEINS

- Beef
- Lamb
- Pork (including reasonable servings of bacon and sausage)
- Poultry (chicken and turkey), preferably free-range and organically fed
- Seafood (wild-caught fish and shellfish; be aware of heavy metal contamination)
- Wild-game meats
- Organ meats
- Eggs (farm-raised and organic; or at least choose those that are high in omega-3s)
- Dairy
- Protein powders (preferably non-dairy and with fewer than five grams of glutamine per serving)

DAIRY PRODUCTS

- Butter (including ghee and clarified butter)
- Full-fat cream cheese (again, look for fillers, including whey protein)
- Some types of hard or ripened cheeses (one ounce or less per serving; count the protein as well)

NUTS AND SEEDS

- Almonds (including almond butter)

- Brazil nuts (rich in selenium but no more than two nuts per day; more is not better)
- Coconut (including coconut cream and unsweetened coconut meat)
- Macadamias (high in good fats; low in carbs and protein; low in oxalates; limit to five to eight per day since they are fattening)
- Pecans (high in fats; low in carbs)
- Walnuts (great for the brain! Put it in your salad. Fewer omega-6s than most nuts)
- Chia seeds (great source of healthy omega-3s and fiber; keep refrigerated)
- Hemp hearts/seeds (great source of healthy omega-3s and complete protein)
- Flaxseed (great source healthy omega-3s and fiber; grind and put in the refrigerator)
- Cashews, cashew butter (use sparingly as these can be fattening)
- Tahini
- Sesame seeds
- Pumpkin seeds
- Pistachios
- Pine nuts
- Hazelnuts

WHOLE GRAINS AND BREADS

- Barley

- Whole grains
- Rice bran
- Pumpernickel bread

FATS AND OILS

- Organic butter or ghee (buy the highest quality you can afford, preferably made from grass-fed animals living on organic and sustainably maintained pastureland)
- Organic coconut, MCT oil
- Omega-3 fish oil, either as fresh fish, or krill oil
- Omega-3 oil from non-animal sources (flax, chia, hemp)
- Organic, cold-pressed, extra virgin olive oil
- Organic avocado and macadamia nut oils (high in monounsaturated fat)

BEVERAGES

- Cold-pressed green juice without any fruits
- Chamomile tea
- Mint tea
- Green tea
- Jasmine tea
- Oolong tea
- Sencha green tea
- Coffee
- Raw apple cider

Appendix D

FOOD SHELF LIFE

By paying attention to the shelf life of your food, you can make sure to eat produce while it is fresh and most nutrient dense.

STORED IN THE REFRIGERATOR

- Apples: 2 weeks
- Blackberries: 2 days stored with a single layer of paper towel
- Blueberries: 1 week
- Bok Choy: 5 days
- Broccoli: 5 days
- Cabbage: 2 weeks
- Carrots: 3 weeks
- Celery: 1 week
- Chard: 4 days
- Endive: 1 week
- French beans: 1 week

- Ginger: 3 weeks
- Lemon: 4 weeks
- Lettuce: 4 days
- Mushrooms: 5 days stored in a paper bag
- Peas (fresh): 5 days
- Pomegranate (seeds): 5 days
- Radicchio: 4 days
- Raspberries: 3 days stored with a single layer of paper towel
- Spinach: 1 week
- Strawberries: 3–4 days stored with a single layer of paper towel
- Zucchini: 1 week

STORED IN THE PANTRY

- Beans (dried): 2 years maximum
- Black pepper: 3 years maximum
- Black teas: 2 years maximum
- Canned tomatoes: 1 year maximum
- Capers (sealed): 1 year maximum
- Chile paste: 1 year maximum
- Coffee (ground): 3 months
- Dried fruits: 1 year maximum
- Dried mushrooms: 1 year maximum
- Dried Spices: 2 years maximum
- Extra virgin olive oil: 6 months
- Garlic: 2 months

- Green teas: 1 year maximum
- Miso paste: 1 year; 6 months after opening
- Nuts: 6 months
- Onions: 1 month
- Pine nuts: 2 months
- Seeds: 3 months
- Shallots: 3 weeks
- Vinegar: 6 years maximum
- Whole grains: 6 months

ACKNOWLEDGMENTS

I would like to thank, first and foremost, **God**, for His never-ending grace. Thank you for believing in my strength and gifting me with a positive mindset to interpret a cancer diagnosis as the best thing that has happened to me. You knew I would be tenacious enough to accept this challenge. With your never-ending guidance and grace, you showed me the importance of loving and prioritizing myself so that I can now turn around and help other people in their health journeys.

Thank you for the belief that gives me an open and generous heart so I can make it my purpose in life to give other cancer patients hope that they, too, do not need to die from this devastating disease. Thank you for giving me the gift of a new life, which is built on an indestructible foundation with one of the most important missions: to give hope to cancer patients that a cancer diagnosis can indeed be a blessing. It is also my mission to wake up the rest of the world, people who are sleepwalking through life, by opening their eyes to living a joyful and meaningful life by embracing a healthy lifestyle that helps prevent disease.

Writing my story would not have been possible without the help and support of many people.

A sincere thanks to **my publishing company**, whom I am thrilled to have as a part of my journey. A special thanks to **Lauren**, who heard my voice and felt my emotions. Thank you for giving me a safe space for those moments when I broke down, showing so much compassion, and understanding that re-living my story is a difficult thing to do. It was a lot of hard work, weekly meetings, and deadlines, but WE did it, Lauren. I appreciate you.

I found my angels in the City of Angels!

The completion of this book could not have been possible without my assistant, **Edward**, who was God sent to me. Initially, I hired him to do some administrative work, including typing my handwritten manuscript. Five minutes after his arrival, he asked me what I do, because he saw that I had a lot of books on health and spirituality, and everything in my kitchen was super healthy. I told him I am a health coach, and that I was writing a book about my cancer journey. He then told me how he is an engineer but would like to eventually change careers and enter the health business. I told him that his God must really love him because he connected us. I told him that I am the perfect mentor and person to work for since I actually walk the talk as a health coach. After ten minutes of typing my handwritten manuscript, he seemed overwhelmed and said, "Your story is crazy! I want to work for you and help you get this book out, and I am willing to do this without pay because I can already tell I can learn so much from your story and being around you!" I thought, *a computer engineer to help a technology inept person like me? How perfect is this!*

"Wow, another grace from God!" From that day onward, Edward has been coming to my home after a full day of work and typing my manuscript. He stays until ten o'clock in the evening during the week and works long hours on the weekend. Edward, I would like to acknowledge you with immense gratitude for the support, the loyalty, and the dedication you have given to me and *The Grace of Cancer.* I met all my deadlines because you consistently showed up and helped me in all phases of writing this book. You are already an amazing young man, and I feel privileged and excited to be working together with you!

In 2017, a year after receiving the cancer diagnosis, another grace from God led me to attend **Carolyn Myss**'s seminar in San Diego. This was my first experience with spirituality and medical intuition. Carolyn Myss asked me to sit with her during a break. She told me that she felt I had a story, and she wanted to hear it. After I shared my story with her, Carolyn told me that it is my responsibility to write a book and to share my story, as I am meant to help people with their cancer journey. Carolyn Myss, thank you for introducing me to spirituality, elevating my consciousness, almost forcefully telling me to write my book, and finally, bringing awareness to the idea that there is grace in getting this disease.

I thank **everyone I know and have not met who has prayed for me** after hearing my diagnosis. I felt your prayers, and God has heard them as well.

My loving family and relatives who are very religious and go to church weekly. I love you for all your support and for understanding that I had to get physically stronger before I could see you. Seeing me in my weakest condition would have been incredibly hard and painful for you, so I knew that the best way to support me was by asking you to pray non-stop to God and ask him to take care of me. Thank you for listening to me.

To my babies, Mirabella, Karina, and Stefan. My three treasures in life! I love you so much, and I wanted everything to be perfect for you. Trying to be this perfect mother while my heart was aching was one of the hardest roles I have ever played in my life. I hope one day you will understand that I couldn't just settle because *you*, my darlings, were watching me.

Thank you to **my sisters from Star of the Sea High School** who went to church to light a candle, praying that this disease did not take me away from this beautiful life. I am so touched that you got together to pray on my behalf.

To all **the high school girls I coached in tennis**, who messaged to tell me that their entire high school prayed for me, and shared beautiful, encouraging words like, "Coach V, you got this! We are rooting for you just like you were rooting for us during our matches." All I could think of was, "Wow, my girls remembered me!" Thank you for warming my heart and putting a smile on my face.

To **Mirella and Howard**, who I consider my East Coast parents and who have known me since I was nineteen years old! I knew the news of me having cancer was devastating to you. Howard, thank you for reaching out to everyone to get me *the* best oncologist and care should I have moved to New York for my cancer treatment. The two of you mean the world to me.

Dr. Fung, thank you for believing in me! You knew I wanted to live, BADLY, so I appreciate you giving me hope when the Western doctors gave me a death sentence. Today, you are not only my doctor but also one of my closest friends, and me being alive is our best work of collaboration! We are an awesome team!

Dr. Fung's staff, thank you for taking care of me and having patience for all the times I showed up late for my appointments, and for not judging me when I showed up completely stoned.

Dr. Myers, thank you for not making me feel bad for having such thin and uncooperative veins. I know poking me several times was hard for you. You knew how important my IV treatments were, so giving up on my veins was not an option!

To **Karen,** who knew I missed traveling, and who gave up her first-class seat at the treatment room for me, to make me feel good. Most of all, thank you for making our treatment sessions like going to a comedy show. Boy did we laugh hard! We were two people connected through our illnesses—how magical is that, my dearest friend? YOU, my darling Karen, are THE badass, and you are my heroine! Keep fighting, my dear Karen! I am here for you and for the rest of our LONG lives!

To **Karen** from Juicy Juice, who saved me and educated me on cannabis. Thank you for taking my arms and telling me that I did not have death in my eyes. I do not think you realized you were one of two people who told me I would not die from this disease! You gave me the gift of HOPE! You were clearly one of the angels that God has sent me to deliver that message.

Maara, my cycling friend, thank you for introducing me to Karen from Juicy Juice. I am glad I listened to you when you told me to see her. You have always been good to me, both before my diagnosis and even more so after. I am grateful for your kindness and generosity.

Ken, my darling friend. You got your wish—you can now beat me in tennis! Just kidding! Ken, you are like a protective brother to me, and your mom is one of the best human beings! I thank you for coming to my home and asking me to pray together. This was so special to me and I will never forget it. I know I am here today because you have told every single person in your family to pray for me. I love your heart, my friend!

Samy, the man who made me feel like a goddess even though cancer made me feel so unattractive. You, my darling Samy, were sent to me by God. You rushed to my side the minute you found out about my diagnosis. Your kind and BIG heart made me feel so adored and safe. Thank you for not leaving me alone at night and always making sure I was taking care of myself. I enjoyed all our intellectual and spiritual conversations. Oh yes… and for pushing me to get back on the tennis court and "crack an egg" with my lethal forehand. Great memories that I cherish, my darling Samy!

Sheila and Brian, thank you for being part of my life. You just knew how to make me feel supported and loved. Thank you for understanding what I needed from you both.

Wallace, our first encounter in SF Tennis Club, when I called you another name! Oops! That was hilarious, or at least I thought so. Little did we know, years later, after moving to LA, I would be calling you to help me understand how to not die! I was so happy to have an oncologist as a friend. You saved me from moving to NYC to be treated at Sloan Kettering. Because of you, I found my Western oncologist! Thank you, Mondesire!

To all the thousands of **men from Match.com who messaged me,** especially to one in particular who referred me to my doctor. Thank you all for making me laugh, for sending me lovely emojis of bouquets of flowers, and for all the kind words that brought joy to me on a daily basis. The power of the goodness in people—yet another grace from the Almighty!

Kathy, another person who has known me since I was in my early twenties. You and I witnessed that hummingbird who managed to fly inside your suite on the ninth floor in San Francisco, and we saw it as a sign that I was going to be just fine! Thank you for hugging me and telling me that the hummingbird was *the* sign I prayed for, and that God was telling me I was going to be all right! You are that second person who had given me hope and reassured me that God was watching over me!

Rosie, one of my favorite artists, who stenciled my mantra and my favorite quote on my walls in my sacred home. I look at these walls daily, and it brings me such joy and peace! You are such a beautiful person with the biggest heart and a kind soul. *Grazie mille*, Rosie!

Sheila, my darling, silly best friend. Although you came later in my journey, I am ecstatic to have you in my life in such a HUGE way! I love our commitment to each other to always make time for sacred moments no matter how busy we can get! I love how I am allowed to have other friends, but I have to love you the most! You are one of the craziest women I know, which is why I adore you. Oh yes…your step in LOVE when hubby is not around, and I will always gladly step into this role as YOU are so worth it!

Lauren, I knew when I met you, you were one of a kind. The sister I never had, a very caring one who will do anything to help! You are my angel who has been there for me, my rock when I needed to hear, "You got this V!" Thank you for believing in me, my darling. You were that person who reminded me that I did not have to climb the mountain alone. *You* were coming with me whether I needed you or not! Thank you for teaching me that it is okay to need YOU!

Emily, you are my fierce best friend who will punch anyone who isn't nice to me! Always ready to believe and defend me. You were there from day one. You helped me find comfort in the most uncomfortable times in my life. You always respected me and the decisions I made. You are that special friend who doesn't need daily conversations because we are so connected by our hearts. Nothing is off-limits since the foundation of our friendship is brutal HONESTY! Thank you for being YOU, my precious Emily!

Pete, you are my brother by heart! You have done so much for me. I have made all my doctor appointments because you made sure you came to get me! You asked all the hard questions that you knew I was too afraid or too stoned to ask. I loved all our celebratory lunches after my scan results would show that the tumors were shrinking. Most of all, thank you for reminding me how strong and brave I am, especially when I feel like I am being weak.

Danelle, my darling friend who came to my life at the perfect time. You are just as crazy and passionate about health as I am. I love how we can talk for hours about all the things we are learning from the conferences that we attend together. The best part—I am not the only weirdo who has a bag of supplements that she takes throughout the day!

Robyn and Mikayla, my international angels who are always looking out for what's best for badass V! I am thrilled to have you co-create with me! As I have said to you, once you are with me, there is no leaving *moi*!

Tayla and Jen, God gave you both to me as my adopted daughters in Los Angeles. You have brought joy to my life, and I am so excited to be part of your journey.

Amber and Lucien, your energy speaks to me, and I felt it during Thanksgiving 2018. Thanks to your healing aura, I gave birth to *The Grace of Cancer* shortly after Amber did my card reading and gifted me with a unicorn card. That was a sign too big to ignore! Thanks for reminding me who I am—BOLD and BRAVE! One who goes after her dream. I listened and started writing my book on December 1, 2018. Yes, now I know that I was divinely guided, because it has been a magical experience since then.

Grace and Taraneh, my San Francisco friends who showed up for me when I needed the comfort of old friends. I appreciate your friendship, especially when I could not give much. Thank you.

ABOUT THE AUTHOR

VERONICA VILLANUEVA discovered her "why" after being diagnosed with stage IV cancer in 2016. She knows she is alive today to share grace, blessings, and the lessons that cancer has taught her. Her "incurable" disease gave her the gift of knowing herself, loving herself, and sharing herself with others in a profound way. Through her work as a trained Cordon Bleu chef and certified health coach, Veronica aims to inspire others to embrace a holistic lifestyle built on a commitment to growth, eating healthy foods, taking the time to create memorable moments, and of course, fostering loving relationships. Learn more and connect with Veronica at http://veronicavillanueva.com/.

Made in the USA
Coppell, TX
19 March 2020